PENGUIN BOOKS

THE WAY TO A HEALTHY HEART

Rekha Shetty is professionally qualified as a medical and psychiatric social worker, with academic training in sociology and management. She has been closely involved in programmes for preventive healthcare in corporate offices and with other people for the last seventeen years.

She is the founder of Mindspower, an organization that helps people lead healthier lives by harnessing the powers of the body, mind and soul.

The Way to a Healthy Heart

THE ZERO HEART ATTACK PATH

R EKHA S HETTY

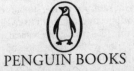

PENGUIN BOOKS

Penguin Books India (P) Ltd., 11 Community Centre, Panchsheel Park,
New Delhi 110 017, India
Penguin Books Ltd., 80 Strand, London WC2R 0RL, UK
Penguin Putnam Inc., 375 Hudson Street, New York, NY 10014, USA
Penguin Books Australia Ltd., 250 Camberwell Road, Camberwell, Victoria
3124, Australia
Penguin Books Canada Ltd., 10 Alcorn Avenue, Suite 300, Toronto,
Ontario, M4V 3B2, Canada
Penguin Books (NZ) Ltd., Cnr Rosedale and Airborne Roads, Albany,
Auckland, New Zealand
Penguin Books (South Africa) (Pty.) Ltd., 24, Sturdee Avenue, Rosebank
2196, South Africa

First published by Penguin Books India 2003

10 9 8 7 6 5 4 3 2 1

Typeset in Charter BT by S.R. Enterprises, New Delhi
Printed at Thomson Press, Noida

While every effort has been made to check the accuracy of all the factual
information contained in the book, the publishers cannot accept responsibility
or liability of any nature whatsoever for any of the said information. Information
and data given along with the opinions and views expressed are those of the
author only.

The medical data is valid at the time of writing. Medicine is an ever-changing
science; therefore new research can change knowledge. These recommendations
are not absolute and should not be construed to apply to all persons.

For my parents Bhoja Shetty and Vinodha Shetty
who taught me, by example, the
Zero Heart Attack Path

CONTENTS

ACKNOWLEDGEMENTS

This book would not have been possible without V.K. Karthika, my empathic and encouraging associate at Penguin.

Poulomi Chatterjee's editorial inputs have made this a better book.

Shubba Shetty's conscientious testing of each recipe in the ZHAP diet plan has made the nutrition section tasty and inspiring. Her support to ZHAP has been valuable and unswerving.

INTRODUCTION

Hari Srivastava was a doctor beloved by all. Exercise was a part of his daily routine. He and his wife would walk in the park for a full forty-five minutes everyday. He ate in moderation, did not touch cigarettes or alcohol and even played tennis regularly. One day at 9 a.m. in the morning, he suddenly dropped dead in the park.

Thirty million people suffer from heart attacks in India every year. Hari was one of the ten million people who die every year within the first five minutes of having a heart attack and do not get time to reach a doctor or a hospital. Ironically, most people are unaware that heart problems can be prevented and even reversed. It is precisely this fact and the waste of life, young and otherwise, which led me to work on the prevention and reversal of heart disease and develop the Zero Heart Attack Path.

What is a coronary heart disease? It takes years for the arteries to get blocked and result in a heart attack. The process takes place silently. 80 per cent of your heart could be blocked without your knowing it. Over the years an unhealthy diet, a stressful lifestyle, smoking, coping with the rat race and the deposition of cholesterol and fat eventually block the arteries and cut off blood and oxygen supply to the heart, leading to a heart attack and possibly an early death.

Inspired by an encounter with an Indian *sanyasi*, Dr Dean Ornish, an American physician, had begun a landmark experiment on reversing heart disease twenty years ago. He proved scientifically that the human heart can repair itself. The ZHAP is based on similar principles to prevent heart disease.

Those who have adopted the ZHAP have begun to feel better right away. They have gained a new understanding of what makes them happy, a calmer attitude, higher energy levels, reduction in blood pressure, decreased chest pain and an overall sense of well-being.

The Way to a Healthy Heart begins by discussing how the heart functions under normal conditions and the factors, both internal and external, that affect its working.

Here you will learn that it is your responsibility to protect your heart. You can keep your heart healthy by being proactive and making sweeping changes in your lifestyle. The book also answers questions on how to increase your happiness quotient, what exercises to perform, happiness and well-being strategies and what to eat in a ZHAP diet.

Indians are genetically more prone to the risk of heart attacks. Today, a fatal heart attack can strike a thirty-year-old. Now is the time to prevent or reverse the disease, for tomorrow may be too late.

Chapter 1

UNDERSTANDING THE HEART

The heart is the engine of life. It supplies the fuel needed to keep every cell of the body alive. It is the most hardworking part of the human body. The heart continues to beat from the minute it is created in your mother's womb till the last moment of your life.

The heart is approximately the size of your fist. Open your fist and close it. Try doing it as though you were trying to crack a walnut. You will find that you cannot continue for more than a few minutes. Yet your heart works even harder, at the same pace, about one lakh times a day, for the whole of your life without ever stopping to rest. This is because of the special nature of the cardiac muscles. The cardiac muscles contract without any signal from the nervous system. So, it is usually believed that you have no control over your heartbeat, which is a part of an autonomic system. However, as recent research has shown, biofeedback systems can help you slow down your heartbeat. The same effect can be achieved through meditation techniques.

The heart is the pump which controls the circulatory system. It weighs 340 g and is about 15 cm in length and 10 cm wide. Protected by the ribcage and the spine, the pear-shaped heart has four chambers. Each side of the heart has an upper chamber called an atrium and a larger lower

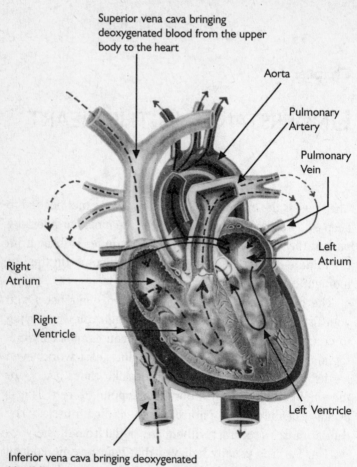

Superior vena cava bringing
deoxygenated blood from the upper
body to the heart

Aorta

Pulmonary
Artery

Pulmonary
Vein

Left
Atrium

Right
Atrium

Right
Ventricle

Left Ventricle

Inferior vena cava bringing deoxygenated
blood from the lower body to the heart

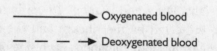

Oxygenated blood

Deoxygenated blood

chamber called a ventricle. There is a one-way valve between each atrium and ventricle which controls the flow of blood from atrium to ventricle. Similar valves also control the flow of blood from the right ventricle to the pulmonary artery and the left ventricle and the aorta. The heart supplies blood to all parts of the body, feeding the cells with oxygen. When the blood has given up its oxygen to the cells, it acquires a bluish tinge and becomes purplish red in colour. The pulmonary arteries or arteries from the lungs carry the deoxygenated blood from the right ventricle of the heart to the lungs, where it once more collects oxygen. The pulmonary veins carry oxygenated blood (blood rich in oxygen) back to the left ventricle of the heart, which pumps the oxygen-rich blood to every cell of your body. It is estimated that the heart pumps blood through 90,000 km of blood vessels everyday.

The normal rate at which the heart of a healthy young adult at rest beats is between 60 to 100 beats per minute. When you exercise, your heart may beat at a rate that is as high as 180 to 200 beats per minute. When you are frightened or excited adrenaline is pumped into the body, causing the heart to beat faster and harder to prepare you for the 'fight or flight' response.

What causes a heart attack?

The two main coronary arteries are the heart's lifelines. They carry oxygen to the heart. They are also the body's lifelines. When they get damaged, serious illness or death is the inevitable result.

The most common disease of the coronary arteries is 'atherosclerosis' or hardening of the arteries. In this disease the tender flexible tissues of the arteries harden and are thickened by the accumulation of fat, thus reducing blood flow through the arteries. When an artery gets blocked by a blood clot and blood cannot flow through it at all, a heart attack occurs, damaging the heart muscle. Those at risk from heart attacks suffer from occasional chest pain. This is known as 'angina pectoris'.

Bypass surgery or angioplasty are usually performed to open blocked arteries. Over 50,000 coronary bypass surgeries are performed every year in the US. These operations entail a lifetime of taking drugs.

Factors that threaten the heart

A pattern is clearly visible among those who are most susceptible to heart disease. Some of these risk factors are out of your hands, but there are many factors that are within your control. You can take decisions that can ensure perfect health for your heart, and a high-quality, long life for you.

Genetic factors

Your family's medical history can give you a clue about the condition of your heart. If there are a number of people in your family who have had heart problems it is an early warning signal that you need to recognize. Remember that you may not show any symptoms even if seventy per cent of your arteries are blocked. Your first symptom could be death.

Stress

Stress is the world's most renowned killer. What is even more important is an individual's response to stress. People have commonly been categorized into two types of personalities. The Type A personality, who is aggressive, ambitious and hyperactive and have a tendency to keep the body in a constant state of high alert, and Type B personalities who are more laid-back and are less liable to respond to stress. It is therefore the Type A personality who is more at risk because of the manner in which he responds to stress.

Sedentary lifestyle

Physical movement has become greatly reduced in today's day-to-day life. Those in the corporate world rarely get an opportunity to engage in physical labour. This reduces respiratory capacity and puts great strain on the cardiovascular system. A life of pushing buttons or riding automobiles can greatly increase the risk of a heart disease. On the other hand, moderate exercise, yoga, or walking for even thirty minutes in a day will reduce that risk. You do not have to be a fitness freak to get results.

Blood pressure

Even a slight increase in blood pressure above the normal 120/80, can affect the functioning of your heart. Anyone whose blood pressure is higher than 140/90 needs to control it. The risk of having a heart attack is at least double for those with hypertension. It is suspected that increased blood pressure damages the walls of the arteries and leads to atherosclerosis. It also reduces the rest periods for the heart.

Cholesterol

Diets that have high fat content are bad for the heart. But even those on a low-fat diet can be affected by heart disease because the liver produces cholesterol as a response to stress, which gets deposited along the inner walls of the blood vessels and affects the functioning of the heart.

Obesity

Those who are overweight by over twenty-five per cent are also at risk. Every extra pound of weight makes the heart work harder. Obesity reduces activity and leads to a vicious cycle of even greater weight gain. Every kilo of excess weight forces the heart to pump blood through an extra 300 km of capillaries!

Smoking

Smoking is an easily avoidable cause of heart disease. The risk of dying due to heart disease shoots up five times for smokers. Smoking increases the formation of blood clots which can cause blockages. Carbon monoxide in the cigarette smoke prevents the blood from carrying the requisite amount of oxygen, forcing the heart to work harder for its supply of oxygen. Smoking causes spasms in the blood vessels even in very young people.

Chapter 2

STRESS THE KILLER

During the Korean War, doctors found that many young men killed in battle had already begun to develop symptoms of heart disease. The unremitting stress of the situation had begun to damage their coronary arteries and the heart. Today's corporate battlefield has the same effect on people. Ambition, increasing peer pressure and rising expectations ensure the rat-in-a-trap syndrome, where people are trapped into running faster and faster to stay in the same place. Jobs are no longer secure and stable. The constant need to upgrade skills to retain a job is challenging and stressful for individuals. Many have to confront the question of how their personal needs and values can be squared with their desire to climb the corporate ladder; this causes serious conflicts in the individual's life.

Work follows us everywhere. The blurring of work and leisure has intensified in this era of twenty-four-hour access—the computer is just a fingertip away and the cellphone is as intimate as a heartbeat. Interactive electronic devices have made stress a constant and overwhelming presence in our lives. Even the home is no longer a refuge. The delicate tissues of the body are constantly submerged in the lethal chemical bath created by chronic stress.

The international information highway and internet fuel the speed of business transactions at the speed of thought, where nano-seconds are critical. We have to constantly rush against the clock and perform many tasks simultaneously. The human body is not wired to be alert round the clock, resulting in intense pressure and stress on the individual.

The personal cost of stress includes burnout, chronic disabling illnesses, crippling tensions in family life, and a loss of personal fulfilment and joy.

The corporate costs of stress are also worth taking into account. From a study of the health records of a well-known US company, it is

---

Physical symptoms of stress

- Breathlessness and palpitations when facing tough situations
- Persistent nausea and vomiting
- Dizziness
- Asthma
- Need to consume alcohol
- Excessive smoking
- Loss of appetite
- Excessive craving for food
- Insomnia
- Nightmares
- Constant fatigue
- Onset of allergies
- Chronic indigestion
- Nail biting
- Constipation or diarrhoea
- Fidgeting
- Frequent headaches or anxiety attacks
- Ulcers
- Becoming accident prone
- Addiction to medication
- Impotence
- High blood pressure
- Anger and incidents of violence

estimated that the annual corporate cost of stress per employee is about US $10,000.

Woman power and how it is affected by stress

Most women in modern societies bear the dual burden of managing the home and a career. However, the infrastructure necessary to help them—crèches, dependable childcare, help from husbands, gadgets to make housework easier—is yet to be firmly established.

Most women face an uneasy acceptance as leaders. There is always an underlying male resentment, which brings in a very stressful factor into the professional lives of senior women executives. These career women also play Supermoms at home and the impact could is extremely damaging for the heart. This generation of transitional women is at high risk from heart disease, particularly during the menopausal years. Statistics show that women have a fifty per cent chance of dying from a heart disease, which is ten times higher than the risk of dying from breast cancer.

The shock absorber of the family, in particularly traditional Indian families, is the woman. Dual responsibilities have reduced her capacity to perform this role. Her ability to absorb and reduce tensions has been greatly compromised. The tensions building up in a nuclear family can have a negative impact on the incidence of heart disease. The two-income family brings an increased pay check, while insidiously increasing the risk factors for heart disease. Huge reserves of patience are required to cope with this new, changed family structure and most people lack these reserves.

As women climb to higher levels of the corporate ladder, alternative strategies have to be found to maintain the nurturing capacity of the family. Only joint efforts by couples and the involvement of elders and the extended family or community support can adequately fill this gap. This pressure-cooker situation is seldom discussed though it is hazardous to health and lethal for the heart.

How does stress affect the heart?

Any of the five negative emotions—*kama* (lust), *krodha* (anger), *madha* (arrogance), *lobha* (greed), *matsarya* (jealousy)—can flood the body with the chemicals of stress.

Let us consider the most common emotion: anger.

When you are angry thirty-six chemicals rush into the blood. This includes lethal chemicals like adrenaline and histamine. The heart rate, the pulse rate and the rate of breathing shoot up. The body gets ready to 'fight or flee'. Digestion stops. All parts of the brain, except the primitive 'reptilian brain' which the primitive man used for survival, are switched off. Today, this desperate 'May-day' survival response is used frivolously, not to save one's life, but in response to office politics or while driving on the road.

As the blood rushes through the heart during an anger attack, it raises the blood pressure. The sudden force of increased blood flow in an enraged person causes minute tears in the tender fabric of the arteries. Fatty deposits like cholesterol, find a convenient place to park themselves to repair the tears and the 'plaster of Paris' of the body slowly builds up to occlude the artery. Soon the tender flexible artery becomes stiff and hard, preparing the stage for a heart attack.

How then do we cope? How can we be successful without damaging ourselves and those we love? How can we be at peace and be happy and still maintain the pace required by

> ### Life destroying experiences
>
> ■ Fear of losing your job.
> ■ Anxiety about not being able to keep up with your peers.
> ■ Working everyday so long and so hard that you are barely able to think.
> ■ Working in a hostile atmosphere where there is competition.
> ■ Being taken for granted by those you love.
> ■ Betrayal.
> ■ Feeling trapped.
> ■ Feeling abandoned.

the corporate world and modern living in general? What are the skills required to deal creatively with the stress epidemic?

How can you cope with stress?

Meditation and Pranayama

Insurance providers have found that the regular practice of meditation reduces heart-related expense by eighty-seven per cent. Meditation and pranayama provide everyone with a way of reducing the automatic violent reactions to stress. Meditation helps you to control autonomous functions like heartbeat and pulse rate which were earlier thought to be outside your control. It can provide you with a silent room within yourself where you can retreat to be at peace. While you cannot change your job, family

> ### Life enhancing experiences
>
> ■ Reassurance from those who matter.
> ■ Going on a holiday with loved ones.
> ■ Enjoying nature.
> ■ Completing a task to your satisfaction.
> ■ Overcoming obstacles.
> ■ Being loved.
> ■ Doing something anonymously for others.
> ■ Acting courageously.
> ■ Sitting in silence.

or the circumstances in which you live, you can certainly learn postures, breathing techniques, concentration and meditation, which will help you to relax, become more alert physically and mentally and avoid what Daniel Goleman in his book *Emotional Intelligence* calls the 'emotional hijack', a Dr Jekyll-Mr Hyde transformation which involves a normal man turning into a hideous beast when he is overcome by anger.

Replace stress with positive emotions

Negative emotions, such as anxiety, fear, depression, anger, impatience, hostility, aggressiveness or overindulgence of any desire, cause imbalance. Moderation leads to harmony. Merely avoiding negative emotions is not enough. You should consistently cultivate the positive emotions—love, compassion, courage, laughter and wonder—that engender joy.

Religion

Religion, said the communists contemptuously, is the opiate of the masses. But studies have shown that prayer and faith calm the mind and slow down the heart and pulse rate. In fact, religion works as a great stress-buster.

Participate in activities that make you happy

All healthcare systems, including modern medicine, are in agreement that a patient's psychological state has much to do with the healing process. Activities like taking part in a *satsang*, singing a tune you enjoy, dancing for fun or participating in activities with children can make you feel contented. You should also learn to enjoy the gifts of nature, such as rain, flowers, a beautiful sunrise or sunset and the variety of life in the natural world.

Support your spouse

The joint family has crumbled to the onslaughts of urbanization. Restlessness and nuclear families in tandem often create explosive situations. A good marriage is a protective shield against heart attacks. Spouses have to be involved in changing the destructive patterns of behaviour which inevitably lead to the development of heart disease.

Find a job that you love

Professor Mihalyi Csikzent speaks about a state called 'flow' which athletes, musicians, surgeons and others experience when they are at their best. It is the experience of being completely involved in whatever you do. So absorbed are you in what you are doing, that there is no place for anxiety or niggling worries in your mind. A job well done also brings with it a certain amount of satisfaction and an immediate increase in self-esteem.

Be unique

In modern corporations there is place only for the contributing members of a team. Restructuring, re-engineering and shrinking profit margins have made the work place increasingly intolerant of unskilled and non-performing members. The only defence against the pink slip is personal excellence and constant growth. This can put a lot of pressure on individuals. Since flatter organizations celebrate individual performance, there is no place to hide in the crowd. While this can be a challenge, constant competition with peers can also be very stressful and exhausting. The only way out is to be unique and innovative.

Chapter 3

THE NAVA RASAS AND THEIR IMPACT ON THE HEART

The concept of 'nava rasas', or nine emotions, is 2000 years old.

Rasa is an emotion. According to the *Natyashastra*, an authoritative treatise on performing arts authored by Bharatmuni, these rasas are: *sringara* (love), *haasya* (laughter), *karuna* (compassion), *vira* (valour), *raudra* (wrath), *adbhuta* (wonder), *bhayanaka* (fear), *beebhatsa* (abhorrence) and *shantha* (serenity).

The human mind is filled with positive and negative emotions. The positive emotions or states like love, laughter, compassion, valour and wonder create a state of happiness and well-being. According to Hinduism and Buddhism, the five negative emotions are lust, anger, arrogance, greed and jealousy. These emotions give rise to restlessness and unhappiness.

The way to a healthy heart lies in nurturing the positive emotions and countering the negative ones.

In order to get the most out of life it is important to be aware of your state of mind.

THE POSITIVE EMOTIONS

Sringara or Love

Sringara is love. Love promotes positive feelings. There are many types of love, ranging from *vatsalya* or mother's love, to *meithri* the love of friends. According to the Greeks, the highest love is platonic love, the pure love between friends. There is also love of the nation, and the universal love and reverence that one feels for all living creatures. Giving and receiving love are both healing and energizing.

———————❖———————

Bring sringara into your life

✓ **Let love come in:** Invite those who love you and those whom you love to enter your life. Reach out for an extended hand and welcome love into your life.

✓ **Give love space and time:** Love needs both quality time and a quantity of time. One cannot replace the other. Leisurely spaces allow love to take root. It flourishes in idleness, in long companionable silences, in tears and in stumbling. Sharing is its life breath.

✓ **Celebrate love:** Celebrate anniversaries and birthdays. Be generous with affirmations. Create occasions to show verbally and non-verbally that you care.

———————❖———————

Haasya or Laughter

Laughter is one of the finest, most economical and easy-to-practice anti-stress measures. A good bout of laughter reduces the levels of stress hormones epineprine and cortisol. When we laugh endorphins and seretonium flow into the blood, resulting in a peaceful, happy state of mind.

Our immune system plays a very important role in maintaining good health and keeping away infections, allergies and cancers. It has been proved by psychoneuroimmunologists that negative emotions like anxiety, depression or anger weaken the immune system of the body, thereby reducing its capacity to fight against infections. According to Dr Lee S. Berk from Loma Linda University, California, USA, laughter helps to increase the count of natural killer cells, a type of white blood cells, and also raises the antibody levels. Researchers have found that laughter therapy causes an increase in antibodies (Immunoglobulin) in those suffering from asthma and bronchitis. Members of Laughter Clubs have actually noticed a decrease in the frequency of common colds, sore throats and chest infections. The effect of laughter on our immune system is considered to be very significant with regard to fatal diseases such as AIDS and cancer.

———— ❖ ————

Introduce laughter into your life

✓ Watch films and television features that make you laugh.

✓ Spend time with cheerful people. Avoid the Cassandras and Agony Uncles.

✓ Avoid toxic people.

✓ Read and share jokes on the internet.

✓ Smile. Do not smother laughter.

✓ Play with babies; make them giggle and laugh with them.

✓ Listen to laughter in a school playground.

———— ❖ ————

One benefit almost everybody derives from laughter is a sense of well-being. The reason for the sense of well-being is that you inhale more oxygen while laughing. Laughter is also one of the best muscle relaxants. According to Dr William Fry from Stanford University, one minute of laughter is equal to ten minutes on the rowing machine. In other words, laughter stimulates heart and blood circulation equivalent to any other standard aerobic exercise. Exercise through laughter is particularly suitable for people who are confined to the bed or to a wheel chair.

Stress is one of the major causes for high blood pressure and heart disease. Laughter helps to control blood pressure by reducing the release of stress related hormones and helping the body and the mind to relax. It has been proved through experiments that there is a drop of 10 to 20 mm pressure after participating for ten minutes in a laughter session.

This does not mean that those with high blood pressure will be completely cured. But laughter definitely helps control and arrest further progress of the disease. Those who are suffering from heart disease and are on medication

---------- ❖ ----------

Have courage

- ✓ Do not be cast down by failure.
- ✓ Enjoy the thrill of overcoming obstacles.
- ✓ Get involved in solving community problems.
- ✓ Resist evil and speak up against injustice.
- ✓ Remember that problems that seem insurmountable are often not so. Approach life with confidence and courage.

---------- ❖ ----------

will find that laughter improves the blood circulation and oxygen supply to the heart muscles. Due to improvement of blood circulation there are less chances of formation of a clot. Those who have had heart attacks or have undergone bypass surgery can also participate in laughter therapy.

Laughter increases the levels of endorphins in our bodies, which are natural painkillers. Norman Cousins, an American journalist who was suffering from an incurable disease of the spine, benefited greatly from laughter therapy when no painkiller could help him. Endorphins released as a result of laughter may help in reducing the intensity of pain in those suffering from arthritis, spondylitis and muscular spasms of the body. Many women have reported a reduced frequency of migraines and headaches resulting from tension after going through laughter therapy sessions.

Karuna or Compassion

Compassion helps create a positive mental state and gets the feel-good chemicals to circulate within you. When you show compassion, the gift you receive is happiness. The Buddhists speak of 'metta bhavana' which means feeling the joy of other living creatures in your being. That is why in pranic healing or reiki or even in organized religions we pray for the peace and happiness of all beings in the universe.

Sharing, helping others and building strong social relationships revv up the immune system, keep us healthy and contribute towards a peaceful life. The presence of pets in cancer wards have been found to hasten the healing process and reduce the negative response to chemotherapy. Studies have shown that those who have four to six close relationships are healthier than those who have less than four. We need social relationships to promote compassion and mutual empathy.

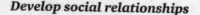

Develop social relationships

- ✓ Take up a sport.
- ✓ Take up a hobby.
- ✓ Volunteer to work for a cause.
- ✓ Join an association in your community.
- ✓ Get involved in your spiritual community.
- ✓ Reach out to someone today.
- ✓ Organize a family get-together.
- ✓ Reaffirm family traditions.
- ✓ Eat together.
- ✓ Give your child a hug.
- ✓ Join or establish self-help groups.

Vira or Valour

Among the nava rasas, valour is essential to the life of a warrior, be it in the battlefield or in the corporate world. Energy, enthusiasm, perseverance, optimism, presence of mind and kindness combine to produce this emotion.

Valour does not just refer to bravery in war. It is the courage that each of us is called upon to manifest in the face of obstacles. The ability to sacrifice, which is the core of emotional intelligence, is integral to vira rasa as is the ability to persist in the face of difficulties, and to face up to the jealousy and pettiness of the world with gentleness, humour and fearlessness. Brilliance and elegance belong to the true warrior who aligns himself with the powerful forces of goodness.

Adbhuta or Wonder

Welcome wonder into your life with a childlike simplicity. Celebrate the beauty of the stars, enjoy the beauty of the mountains, greet the dawn and watch the sunset. Inhale fresh air with deep breaths and contemplate on the creation of the world, the variety in nature that has the capacity to heal you physically and emotionally, the people around you and the everyday human relationships that make all the difference in your life.

Appreciate the wonder in life

- ✓ Be alone in silence at the beginning and end of each day.

- ✓ Enjoy a walk among tall trees and green gardens.

- ✓ Plant seeds and trees; distribute them to people you know.

- ✓ Set apart time for prayer to praise God for his glorious creation.

- ✓ Set apart time to enjoy the beauty in nature and in human beings.

THE NEGATIVE EMOTIONS

Bhayanaka or Fear

Fear is a negative energy. Unless you confront it, it follows you everywhere like a shadow. Fear and its product, anxiety, cause your courage to leak out of the system and result in an inability to act. It fills the body with stress and traps the mind into being depressed and indulging in negative thoughts.

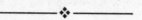

Overcome fear

- ✓ Believe in yourself and your actions.

- ✓ Confront your fear. Think of all the possible consequences of your fear coming true. Rationalize the situation and you will find that things are never as bad as they seem.

- ✓ Do not be afraid of failure. It is just another experience to learn from.

Raudra or Anger

People with hostile personalities have five times the death rate before the age of fifty than people who are less prone to anger. According to Cleyer Freidman, a cardiologist, constant pressure to race against time causes hostility and a sense of insecurity fuels this feeling.

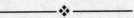

Deal with anger

Red light

- ✓ Stop, calm down and think before you act.

Yellow Light

- ✓ State the problem to yourself and think hard over how you feel about it.

- ✓ Set a positive goal.

- ✓ Think of all the possible solutions.

- ✓ Think ahead about the consequences.

Green light

- ✓ Go ahead and try the best plan.

Beebhatsa or Abhorrence

Disgust and hatred of anything characterize this emotion. It fills you with negativity and an obsession with the object or person that you hate.

Banish hatered

- ✓ Acknowledge feelings of disgust and retreat from them as rapidly as possible.

- ✓ Try to cultivate indifference towards the event or person.

- ✓ Try to avoid the people or situations that arouse this emotion in you till you can become indifferent.

Surround yourself with positive people. Imagine you are a lovely glass jug. Be with people who can pour in words, feelings and thoughts that are clean and beautiful. Stay away from those who pour in poisons and toxins, who constantly make you angry and irritable. Avoid them, because they have nothing to give you but can diminish your happiness and affect your heart like a thousand poisoned arrows.

Chapter 4

THE THREE-WAY PATH TO A HEALTHY HEART

The Three-Way Path

The first step towards attaining a sense of complete harmony that encompasses your whole being is to detoxify

	BODY	MIND	SPIRIT
Detoxify	Do not consume anything that will not enhance your well-being or health.	Avoid people who induce negative thoughts in you.	Rid your mind of all unhappy thoughts as soon as you wake up in the morning.
	Give up smoking and alcohol. Eat fatty foods and sweets in modernation.	Avoid situations that draw you into a field poisoned with arrogance, greed or jealousy.	Forgive those who have harmed you.
		Live one day at a time. Enjoy it.	Wash away all the thoughts that depress you.
		Write down all that worries you and hand it over to God for his help.	Sit in silence.

yourself. Detoxification means emptying your body, mind and soul of all the things that distress you.

But detoxification is not enough. You will need to rejuvenate and heal yourself.

	BODY	**MIND**	**SPIRIT**
Rejuvenate	Eat high energy, high quality, fresh food to increase *prana* or the universal life force within you.	Read books that are elevating and inspiring, and capable of generating creative ideas.	Concentrate on your breathing.
	Exercise moderately.	Meditate twice a day.	Visit a holy place once a week.
	Sleep well. Rest when you are tired.	Interact with people who are positive and encouraging.	Set apart time to read a spiritual book and reflect on your day.
	Invest in a weekly oil bath.	Seek the company of fine thinkers.	Pray to God as you experience him.
		Volunteer to be part of groups which help others and build a network of friends.	

The Rule of Three

Love yourself

To love yourself you must learn to accept yourself as you are. Focus on your skills and talents and develop them. Affirm and celebrate these qualities. Forget what you are not good at. Nothing was ever built on what someone cannot do!

Professor Howard Gardner, in his landmark work on multiple intelligence, says that everyone has atleast one of the seven types of intelligence:

Logical mathematical intelligence, or the capacity to think logically;

Musical intelligence, or the capacity to understand sound and harmony which often emerges very early in life;

Linguistic intelligence, or a mastery over words and the capacity to speak and write well;

Visual spatial intelligence, or excellence in visual forms in space, such as inventors, sculptors, architects;

Kineasthetic intelligence, or the perfect coordination of the body and mind seen in great sportsmen or skilled surgeons;

Knowledge of self, and *knowledge of others*, which is the intelligence that charismatic leaders like Gandhiji possessed.

Take time to identify your own portfolio of intelligences. Use your resources to expand and develop what God has bequeathed upon you. Remember it is important if not crucial to nurture your strengths. Native intelligence is like a seed. If a seed is wrapped in a piece of paper and left in a drawer, forgotten, it will be eaten by ants and reduced to nothing. But a seed which is planted in the warm earth braves storms and challenges to grow into a plant or a tree, which in its turn will bring forth millions of seeds. Similarly, your talents need to be nurtured if they are to flower. If they are ignored they will die.

Love others

Loving others is healing, nourishing and rejuvenating. You can create a magic circle around your loved ones, your home or your office and fill that imaginary circle with kind words and loving and thoughtful gestures. The positive nurturing quality of that circle will sweep away tensions, anger, anxiety and fear.

Those who doubt this, should read Norman Cousins' *The Anatomy of an Illness*. It tells the story of a man nearing death, who cured himself through laughter, happiness and by being in the company of loving friends. He retreated from a stressful job and immersed himself in a life that was joyous and nurturing. In short, he recreated a healthy body through an attitude transplant.

All of us see ourselves through the eyes of the people who are important to us. That is why when we fall in love, we suddenly find ourselves more beautiful, capable and brilliant. This is the image of ourselves that we see reflected in the eyes of the beloved. By loving someone we get the opportunity to encourage another person to achieve his or her full potential.

When human beings love others, or devote themselves to a cause higher than themselves, they recreate for themselves and others, the chemistry of well-being or good health.

'Service is the rent you pay for your room on earth' says an ancient Arabic proverb. Service and caring for others is probably the easiest way to immunize yourself against heart attacks and reverse a heart disease.

A research conducted at the Harvard School of Psychology studied the immune systems of students before and after they had watched a film that showed Mother Teresa ministering to the sick and dying. The blood chemistry of those who watched the Mother showed a marked enhancement in immune response. If just watching a film about kindness can do this to you, imagine what actually serving others could achieve. Develop your capacity to enjoy the happiness of other creatures. If you can enjoy the joy of others, you have a source of eternal, unending joy. While it may be difficult to constantly find joy in the happiness of others.

Love learning

Learning is to the mind and the spirit what food is to the body. Research has proved that learning something new, stretching your mind beyond its natural limits results in new neural connections in the brain well into old age. Such people are far less likely to develop Alzhiemer's disease. Even an activity as simple as solving a crossword regularly can accomplish this.

We can learn from every event in life, not just from what we read in books. This is exemplified in the story about Krishna and Uddhava—

Uddhava, in the course of discussing the mysteries of life with his friend Krishna, asks him, 'Who is a Guru or a teacher?' Krishna says, 'Look at the sky. There is a beautiful strong eagle flying miles above in the sky. However, in a single moment, it can swoop down to earth and pick up its prey. As far as vision is concerned that eagle is your guru. See the lion in the forest, how regal is its gait. As far as physical grace is concerned, that lion is your guru. See the serpent in the jungle, which stands and waits for its prey, confident that nature will provide. As far as confidence in life is concerned, that serpent is your guru. All the events and people in your life are there to teach you something. You can learn something from those you love. You can learn more from those you hate. Life is the great textbook uniquely designed for each person according to his learning needs. Life is the ultimate guru. Whether or not you want to learn from it depends on you.'

Books and films present an opportunity to share others' experiences. Choose those that will enhance your understanding and happiness. Do not introduce into your mind anything that will make you afraid or anxious or sad for too long.

Choose your friends carefully. There is no doubt that everyone can teach you something. But there are many things you do not really need to learn. When you find that someone is spreading gloom, negativity and unhappiness in your life, run! If this person is an inseparable part of your life, try to get the person to be affirmative and positive. Sometimes this can be a real challenge, particularly if this person is very close to you.

Be in touch with all the wonderful things happening around you. Sensitize yourself to the beauty of people, events and nature.

Chapter 5

THE HAPPINESS QUOTIENT AND EMOTIONAL FIELDS

The Happiness Quotient

Your personal Happiness Quotient (HQ) is a measure of your capacity to fill the mind with positive emotions and the ability to deal constructively with negative emotions and eliminate them.

When you are happy chemicals like seretonin and endorphins which fill you with a sense of peace and happiness flood the body. When your HQ is high, your breathing is slow and the heart rate and pulse rate are steady, the mind is calm and alert, digestion is perfect and the food is easily and quickly transformed into energy that the body uses to regenerate and repair the body.

It is not enough to get rid of negative emotions in order to increase your HQ . Your mind is like the land around your home. If the land is full of rocks, snakes, poisonous insects and thorns, that is, negative emotions, then getting rid of them will help; but this will leave behind arid space, which will not give you comfort or joy. If you want a garden you will have to plant beautiful flowers, ferns and creepers. You will have to fill your mind with positive emotions which will bring joy into your life.

How can you increase your HQ?

Know yourself

Be loving and kind to yourself. Speak to yourself as you would speak to your beloved or your child. Treat your body and your mind gently and affectionately with love and understanding.

Sit in silence. Close your eyes and think about your body as full of health and energy. Listen carefully to your breathing and the beating of your heart. As your mind gradually becomes peaceful and tranquil, you will begin to notice the destructive effects of stress. You will become aware of the first, imperceptible symptoms: the tightening of the jaw, the clenching of muscles in your throat and abdomen, the acceleration of the heartbeat. Once you are aware of the symptoms you can consciously control.

Alcoholics Anonymous has a four letter word that describes the sensations that have to be handled: HALT. They say don't be too Hungry, too Angry, too Lonely or too Tired. If you are able to handle or prevent these four states of being, then you will not be swept into actions you will regret later. The capacity to control and soothe yourself, as one would handle a frightened horse or a hysterical child, is a skill that is necessary to cope competently with loss, failure or distress.

A high level of tolerance when faced with frustration flows out of a capacity to motivate oneself. The capacity to sacrifice, to wait and not rush to gratify every desire are skills in this area. Young Siddhartha, the protagonist in Herman Hesse's book of the same name, describes these skills when he to talks to his prospective employer Kumaraswamy. Kumaraswamy asks him, 'What do you know that I should give you a job?' Siddartha says, 'I can wait, I can fast, I can pray.' He gets the job and proves to be a great success at it.

Know others

A drug addict once explained the difference between sympathy and empathy. He said, 'You can never feel anything but sympathy for me and what I need is empathy. Empathy is the capacity to feel my pain in your heart.' Develop the capacity to pick up subtle verbal, tonal and non-verbal signals from others. To be what Peter Salovey calls 'socially tone-deaf' can lead to a life littered with broken relationships. Learn also the ability to send out soothing, nurturing signals to people around you, thus creating a positive interpersonal field.

Unlike in a magnetic field, where positive attracts negative and vice versa, a positive emotional field attracts positive people and events, and in addition, even transforms a person who normally has a negative mindset into a person who thinks positively. Those who can create positive fields around themselves attract and build enduring relationships. The skill of handling conflicts effectively is part of the package. Effective leadership is built on the foundation of this skill. To soothe the anxiety of others, to make them feel comfortable, to build their self-esteem and to encourage them to build on their strengths is at the very heart of leadership. Learn to create a positive field around your home, your office and your life.

The Positive Field

Learning to create a positive field is an important part of Zero Heart Attack Path (ZHAP). The positive field is created by certain tools and models of behaviour, which may be verbal, tonal or non-verbal.

- *Ping pong:* Foremost among the tools is ping pong. In ping pong, every idea is kept in the air as long as possible. The idea is developed by a constant endeavour to isolate its positive aspects and build on them. The more facile a thinker, the more adept he is at discovering the spark of value in the mass of unusable thoughts that is part of the germinal thinking process. The challenge is to keep the thought in the air as long as possible.
- *Community activities:* The positive field is created by a common prayer or mantra, by a mental process which draws a magic circle around all those who are participating. A group activity, a company song, common goals, all enhance the power of the positive field. A handshake, a friendly look, an encouraging word are key factors that widen the positive field.
- *Laughter:* The role of laughter, generated by commonly shared jokes, is vital in creating a positive field.
- *Affirmations:* According to George Prince, the founder of Synectics, a company dealing specifically with creativity and innovation, the most important constituents of the positive field, are affirmations. An affirmation is a verbal, tonal or non-verbal act of appreciation. A compliment can be a verbal hug. A hug can replace a thousand words.

A Sanskrit verse says: 'Don't speak harsh words. If you have to say something unpleasant, do it as kindly as possible while genuinely appreciating the good qualities of the person and the relationship.'

The great Tamil poet, Thiruvalluvar expressed it succinctly when he said, 'Why speak harsh words when kind words are available? Who would eat bitter, unripe fruit when sweet ripe fruits are at hand?' When harsh words are spoken or undesirable events occur, do not allow them to take root like evil weeds. Sweep them away and search for the gentle kindness that lies beneath this harsh exterior.

- **Prana:** *Prana* is the life force that flows in all living things. When the life force leaves the body, it dies. When *prana* is in full flow, the person is full of vitality, energy and enthusiasm. It enhances the positive field.

  Prana is nurtured by freshly cooked, healthy food. It is nourished by breathing in pure fresh air. Pranayama and yoga help to develop the life force. Meditation and a calm attitude enable prana to flow smoothly through all our activities.

  Getting too hungry or eating too much, consuming stale food, exercising till you are ready to drop dead, constant arguments, over-working, getting upset, breathing polluted air, all interfere with the smooth flow of *prana*. Moderation in all things is of the essence.

Ojas and Tejas

According to an ancient Indian belief 'ojas' is the dazzling, vital life force in all living things. If you see a fruit freshly plucked from a tree it is full of ojas. A child playing cricket with complete josh is full of ojas. Sunlight is ojas. A plant burgeoning with green shoots and flowers, is full of ojas. Pure air, the earth, rivers, fresh water, freshly cooked food are all full of ojas. If you consciously approach your body, mind and soul reverently to fill it with ojas, you will enjoy vibrant, vital, good health.

Ojas fills you with 'tejas' which is the dazzling splendour that shines forth from one who celebrates ojas like the ancient rishis. Invite ojas into your life to keep your heart healthy.

HOW A POSITIVE FIELD IS CREATED

Attitudes

Appreciative

Supportive

Respectful

Non-violent

Believing in win-win solutions

Trusting and open

Interested

Optimistic

Willing to share responsibility

Recognizing the value in others' ideas

Understanding others before seeking to be understood

Treating as an equal

Knowing that no task is impossible

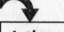

Actions

Show unconditional positive regard

Pray together

Sing together

Exercise together

Practise yoga and meditation

Listen attentively

Show interest

Show approval

Provide support

Protect vulnerable beginnings

Verbal and non-verbal expressions

Smile

Hug

Encourage through eye contact and words

Give gifts

Suspend judgement

Postpone reaction

Build new ideas, add value to them

Accept

Embrace

Shake hands

Share jokes

- ***Drala:*** Tibetans of the Shambala tradition believe in a similar concept called *drala*. *Drala* is a space that is sanctified by reverence, purity and faith. When you treat your space in your work place with reverence and keep it clean and sparkling, you attract *drala* into that space. *Drala* makes that space powerful and attractive. When you dress carefully and concentrate on how you speak and behave, you attract personal *drala*.

Many people are able to do this within their homes. Most Indian homes have beautiful white patterns drawn at the entrance to their homes to attract the goddess of good fortune. The atmosphere is further enhanced by the fragrance of incense and joss sticks. Certain mantras or the sound of bells or wind chimes in a Chinese home are said to purify the atmosphere.

When you consider yourself as sacred, you will treat yourself well. You will wear clean clothes. You will smile at yourself, encourage yourself. In the same way you will clean up the mental space or field around you. You will sweep out all ill will, anger, fear and anxiety. You will accept into that field only what is bright and elevating, fine and happy. The space around you, your house and your office need the same kind of careful attention.

Try to approach all events and all people with affection and reverence. This reverence is due to all because of the divine spark that dwells in all men whether he is a legend or a leper. Sometimes this divine spark is obvious. It is the silent flame of consciousness that reaches out to you from a flowering creeper or your pet. Sometimes this life force loses its vitality and gets dimmed by lethargy and lack of care. Always make sure that the life force is alive in you.

- **The springboard:** The springboard is a tool that can help generate a positive field around you. When someone offers you an idea that may not be too practical or feasible, look for those things in the idea that please you. Thereafter you may say 'Though I like your idea, I have a concern about the cost involved (or time or whatever bothers you). How can we solve it?' In this way you can promote cooperation and collaboration rather than conflict.

The Negative Field

A negative field is characterized by distrust. If you cannot believe in those close to you, you will slowly lose confidence in yourself.

If some people in the group feel excluded they cannot contribute good ideas. They are afraid to think differently and new ideas wither even before they are formulated. They may even change the nature of a positive field by their unhappiness. Just as a drop of cyanide can poison a clear

---

Negative energy

Imagine you are a beautiful transparent glass vase full of pure golden liquid. Now imagine an iron spear crashing into you. That is happens when you allow negative emotions like rage to tear through you. Jealousy is like filling the vase with corrosive poison, which eats away the inside of the vase like acid would. Fear dries up energy causing the glass to crack in the heat which robs you of all energy.

HOW A NEGATIVE FIELD IS CREATED

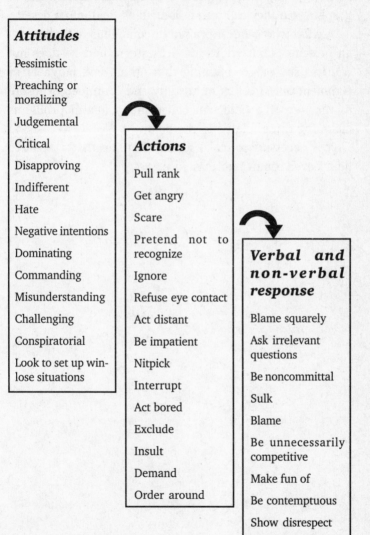

Attitudes

Pessimistic

Preaching or
moralizing

Judgemental

Critical

Disapproving

Indifferent

Hate

Negative intentions

Dominating

Commanding

Misunderstanding

Challenging

Conspiratorial

Look to set up win-
lose situations

Actions

Pull rank

Get angry

Scare

Pretend not to
recognize

Ignore

Refuse eye contact

Act distant

Be impatient

Nitpick

Interrupt

Act bored

Exclude

Insult

Demand

Order around

Verbal and non-verbal response

Blame squarely

Ask irrelevant
questions

Be noncommittal

Sulk

Blame

Be unnecessarily
competitive

Make fun of

Be contemptuous

Show disrespect

Grumble

Threaten

Argue

pool of water, so too the unhappiness of a single person can poison a home or a company. They emanate toxic waves of hostility, and they can turn a flourishing field into a desert.

A child who is never praised or complimented turns into an insecure adult with little self-esteem and he does not want to say or do anything that others will laugh at or comment on. This fear of hostility and continued exposure to the negative field can cause many health problems including those related to the heart.

It is necessary to make sure at all times that a negative field never comes into existence.

Chapter 6

HOW TO IMPROVE YOUR HAPPINESS QUOTIENT

A high HQ is indicative of a healthy heart. You can increase your HQ by filling your mind with positive emotions, events

———— ❖ ————

Increase your HQ

- Do not put yourself down.
- Take pride and pleasure in what you do.
- Do not do things that make you unhappy.
- Consciously do the things that make you happy.
- Do not be unkind to others.
- Do something to make others happy.
- Do what you love; enjoy it.
- Admit to mistakes; try to rectify them.
- Forgive, and let go of resentment.
- Accept responsibility for your life.
- Use your time fully and in a way that pleases you.
- Enjoy the child in you.
- Growth is painful and adventure is risky, but it's worth it.
- Enjoy the moment; forget the past.
- Learn to soothe yourself when you are hurt.
- Soothe others who are hurt.

———— ❖ ————

and people. You should learn to create a positive field around yourself, your home and your workplace.

Physical Health

Your HQ is instantly affected by your physical condition. It is very difficult to be energetic and enthusiastic if you are not in good health. The absence of disease is no indication of a state of perfect health. According to the ancient Indian physician Sushruta, a person is considered to be in perfect health when all parts of his body are functioning perfectly— a body which digests food, feels, moves and acts perfectly— and when his 'body, mind and spirit remain full of bliss'. He focusses on the fluid functioning of a person who knows the perfect balance of body, mind and soul.

Just as you would not tolerate a minor malfunction in your car, so too, you and your doctor should look out for the slightest disturbance in your state of health. Minor problems, aches and pains should be dealt with immediately, rather than endured with gritted teeth.

Listen to your body. If you are tired, rest. If you are hungry, eat. If you are lonely, communicate, ask for a hug. If you are angry, deal with your anger constructively and resolve it.

Choose the fuel for rebuilding your body with care. Sit down peacefully to eat. Close your eyes and rid your mind of all other thoughts; just concentrate on the food before you. Thank the universe for creating the food that will give you the energy to accomplish your goals. Focus on the sight of the food, the smell, the feel and finally the taste. As you chew remind yourself constantly that the food you are eating is responsible for repairing and nourishing all the cells in your body.

The body is our vehicle to act in this world. It has to be kept in good condition so that we may achieve the goals for which we were created. There are many steps to achieve perfect health.

The quiz given below will help you to mentally consider your physical condition. A complete medical check-up once a year can provide accurate information about your heart's condition to your cardiologist.

 Ask yourself

	Yes	No	?
Is good physical health important to me?	☐	☐	☐
Do I pay enough attention to exercise and diet?	☐	☐	☐
Can I honestly say that I exercise on a regular basis?	☐	☐	☐
Do I set aside a regular time for exercise to help me be more consistent?	☐	☐	☐
Do I have healthy eating habits?	☐	☐	☐
Do I eat in a peaceful environment?	☐	☐	☐
Have I ever smoked tobacco?	☐	☐	☐
Have I ever taken drugs or consumed alcohol?	☐	☐	☐
Am I often overwhelmed by lust, anger, possessiveness, greed and jealousy?	☐	☐	☐
Do I sleep for eight hours?	☐	☐	☐

Is my body alert and energetic at
all times? ☐ ☐ ☐

Do I tend to ignore minor health
disturbances and pains? ☐ ☐ ☐

Do I have regular health check-ups? ☐ ☐ ☐

Do I live among people who are
positive and peaceful? ☐ ☐ ☐

Do I watch TV for five hours or more? ☐ ☐ ☐

Do I travel everywhere by car? ☐ ☐ ☐

Do I eat atleast one hot meal a day? ☐ ☐ ☐

Do I eat breakfast? ☐ ☐ ☐

Score

7 to 11 yeses: Good

You take good care of your physical health. Remember that
your body is like a car given to you to travel through life. Or
as the Buddhists say, like a raft required to cross the river. If
you are wise, you will maintain the car and make sure the
raft is in a good condition.

4 to 6 yeses: Adequate

While you are sensible about your physical health, you have
to listen more closely to the signals. You need to be more
proactive about preventive maintenance. The boat may not
be about to sink, but it certainly has a few leaks that need
to be fixed.

Less than 4 yeses: Poor
You need to take more care of your body, or you will sink!
Enlist the support of your physician. Take it easy!

○ **Affirmations** ○

Sit peacefully and breathe deeply with your eyes shut. As
you concentrate on your body, affirm silently:

- I am growing healthier and more beautiful everyday.

- My body is becoming healthier and stronger.

- The special, tasty, fresh food I eat will fill my body
  with peace and happiness.

- The food I eat will heal my heart.

- I am careful about my body and treat it with love.

- I will eat only what is good for the health and
  well-being of my body.

Mental Health

Your HQ has a direct and obvious connection with your
state of mind. Accept yourself, your body and your mind,
as you are. While trying to improve both, affirm and love
yourself as you are today, in the here and now.

If you do not love yourself, you can never love anyone
else. Support yourself, treat yourself like you would treat
the person you love the most.

You are the mirror, in which all your loved ones see
themselves. You can soothe and inspire them by reflecting
back an image that is lovable and competent. Calvin Cooley,
a renowned sociologist, describes the mirror image thus: 'I

am what I think you think I am'. If you are constantly putting down others, they can be mentally disturbed and their unhappiness can harm you.

Unrealistic expectations about your child can put unrelenting pressure on him. Constant criticism of your spouse can make him or her feel unloved and inadequate. They can then become cranky and difficult.

? **Ask yourself**

	Yes	No	?
Do I keep in touch with my subject through regular reading?	☐	☐	☐
Am I aware of what's happening in the world?	☐	☐	☐
Do I have clear, written goals?	☐	☐	☐
Are my actions geared towards those goals?	☐	☐	☐
When I am angry with others do I keep my feelings to myself?	☐	☐	☐
Do I talk to someone I trust about my anger?	☐	☐	☐
Can I convey my views, even if they are different, without losing control?	☐	☐	☐
Am I in the habit of putting myself down?	☐	☐	☐
Do I have a few close friends who give me unconditional love?	☐	☐	☐
Do I have a problem being alone?	☐	☐	☐
Do I pray or meditate everyday?	☐	☐	☐

Am I often anxious about tasks? ☐ ☐ ☐

When faced with new opportunities and
situations, do I strive to be successful? ☐ ☐ ☐

Do I allow others to give me pictures
of who I am? ☐ ☐ ☐

Do I ever think about or subconsciously
fear competing with people? ☐ ☐ ☐

Should I be more concerned about
competing with myself instead of others? ☐ ☐ ☐

Do I often feel I am under a lot of stress
and pressure? ☐ ☐ ☐

Does this stress reflect my own fears? ☐ ☐ ☐

Do I compare myself with others and
feel jealous? ☐ ☐ ☐

Do I worry about what my bosses think
of me? ☐ ☐ ☐

Do work situations often make me angry? ☐ ☐ ☐

Am I afraid of losing my job or being
overlooked for a promotion? ☐ ☐ ☐

Do I continue to work even if I am
exhausted? ☐ ☐ ☐

Do I stay at my workplace for more
than ten hours? ☐ ☐ ☐

Do I routinely eat my meals late? ☐ ☐ ☐

SCORE

9 to 14 nos: Good
Stress, worry, anxiety and fear are like burdens you carry on your shoulders. You have taken a decision to say no often enough, to lay down those burdens and walk freely, happily through life, with a strong heart.

5 to 8 nos: Adequate
While you are not a worry-wart or overburdened by negative emotions, you need to lighten up. Laugh more, fear less. Worry only robs you of your strength to tackle today's problems.

Less than 5 nos: Poor
You need to halt. Take stock. Your heart is in serious danger. Review the past and take decisions for a worry-free future.

○ Affirmations ○

Sit with your eyes closed and silently affirm:

- The world is a positive and healthy place.

- I am a kind and lovable person.

- God loves me and I am loved by my friends.

- I do my best to make my world a happier and better place.

- I can handle failure because a failure is only an event, not the end of my life.

- I am protected by the goodness and wholeness of the universe.

◆ I can tap into the peace and silence of the universe, which is always available to me.

Social

'No man is an island, entire of itself; every man is a piece of the continent, a part of the main, . . .'

Meditations XVII, John Donne

Man is a social being and his personal intelligence forms the basis of a happy, fulfilling life. Personal intelligence is of two types: intrapersonal and interpersonal. Intrapersonal intelligence is the ability to understand others and to empathize with them. Interpersonal intelligence is the ability to understand oneself, to come to terms with what really is. To those who define success as happiness, these two elements can be the bedrock of a happy life.

There are those who can understand the feelings of others as though they were feeling it. Sensitive people can

Remarks that build enduring relationships	*Remarks that destroy relationships*
❏ I agree.	❏ What I can't stand about you is. . .
❏ I really enjoy talking to you.	❏ Trust you to come up with an impossible idea.
❏ Good job!	
❏ I made a mistake, I'm sorry.	❏ You have no idea about this.
❏ I couldn't do it that well even if I tried.	❏ It sounds O.K., but it is quite impractical.
❏ You're on the right track.	❏ Be serious.
❏ That's a winner of an idea!	❏ Has anyone done it before?
❏ If anyone can do it, you can. I believe in you.	❏ Let's ask somebody else.
	❏ You don't understand our culture.
❏ Congratulations!	
❏ What I really like about you is. . .	❏ Nothing you say works.

empathize with others. Charismatic leaders are able to reach out to others by breaking the barriers that exist between people. A charismatic speaker can get thousands of people to react like one mind.

The basis of social success lies in the ability to build pleasant and harmonious relationships with all. Leadership and popularity are built on the skills of nurturing, building and supporting.

Inclusion and Exclusion

Belonging to a supportive nurturing group is the best protection you can have against a heart attack. Being loved can prevent you from the flood of negative emotions that can engulf your heart. With the breakdown of the joint family more and more people becoming victims of heart disease. You must invest in your family and keep in touch with your extended family.

Being 'included' in a group is very healing. Study the group to which you belong. Stay in it if you

- Have common goals
- Communicate easily
- Share jokes
- Use pet names
- Discuss personal successes and failures
- Spend quality time together
- Pay compliments to each other
- Offer comfort and support

Leave the group immediately if the members

- Constantly criticize
- Never pay compliments
- Speak in secret codes
- Share jokes which you do not understand
- Do not make eye contact
- Constantly tease you
- Do not offer you a seat
- Do not send you invitations to gatherings
- Laugh at your ideas or gang up against you

 Ask yourself

	Yes	No	?
Do I try to create a positive field around me, in my home, at work, in social situations?	☐	☐	☐
Am I friendly with all people—friends and strangers?	☐	☐	☐
Am I sincere in what I say and do?	☐	☐	☐
Do I ever talk destructively about people behind their backs?	☐	☐	☐
Do I pay attention to others' needs?	☐	☐	☐
Do I receive help and support from friends?	☐	☐	☐
Do I need to be more independent?	☐	☐	☐

Is shaking hands or remembering names
important to me?　　　　　　　　☐　☐　☐

Do I like meeting new people?　　☐　☐　☐

Am I too loud, boisterous, and talkative
in the wrong situations?　　　　　☐　☐　☐

Am I too shy and quiet in most situations?　☐　☐　☐

Can I carry on a conversation easily with
others in many different areas of interest?　☐　☐　☐

Do I behave hypocritically or inconsistently?　☐　☐　☐

Do I say I believe in one thing and then
do the opposite?　　　　　　　　☐　☐　☐

Do I keep promises?　　　　　　　☐　☐　☐

Do I concern myself with challenges and
problems? Do I keep in touch with
current events?　　　　　　　　　☐　☐　☐

In certain social situations, do I ever give
verbal support to ethical or moral standards
that are different from what I personally
believe and feel?　　　　　　　　☐　☐　☐

Are there any community organizations that I
would benefit from joining?　　　☐　☐　☐

Am I part of an organization which is toxic?　☐　☐　☐

Do I hate anyone?　　　　　　　☐　☐　☐

Am I able to deal with conflict constructively?　☐　☐　☐

Score

10 to 12 yeses: Good
You are cushioned from life's problems by good, loving, long-term relationships. These relationships stress-proof your heart against disease.

6 to 9 yeses: Adequate
You have helpful people around you, but you need to improve your attitude towards others for a truly supportive community life.

Less than 5 yeses: Poor
The lack of social skills exhibited by this score can be lethal to your heart. Work on your people skills.

○ Affirmations ○

Sit with your eyes closed and affirm silently:

- ◆ I have a harmonious relationship with most of the people I meet.
- ◆ I enjoy the pleasure and happiness of others.
- ◆ I look for what is positive in others.
- ◆ I consider most situations to be learning experiences.
- ◆ I try to make others feel comfortable.
- ◆ Awareness of the need of others to be appreciated is the basis of my relationships.
- ◆ I am sincere.
- ◆ I try to express negative emotions in as non-destructive a way as possible.

- ◆ I will draw a magic circle of love around those who interact with me.

The Workplace

Many of us spend most of our time at work. If we do not enjoy our work or feel overwhelmed by it, the constant pressure of the situation will cause inescapable damage to our arteries and other delicate tissues. It will also slow down the body's capacity to repair this damage.

The break-up of community feelings, urbanization and the highly competitive work culture have increased the possibility of unhealthy workplaces.

'Fast tracking' and trying to be a corporate star will extract the inevitable price of damage to arteries if you are not aware of the impact your actions can have on your body and mind. You must learn to distinguish the state of your body when you are relaxed from the unrest in the system when you are in the clutches of the five negative emotions, *kama*, *krodha*, *madha*, *lobha* and *matsarya*. This awareness will help you unclench and relax the muscles, slow down the racing heart beat by consciously breathing slowly and calmly.

Welcome and embrace active positive emotions. They are the success of life, the secret of health, the foundation of energy. Another way to protect your heart and keep your arteries young could be to work at something you love, to be 'self actualized' in Maslow's terms.

——————— ❖ ———————

Bring harmony into the workplace

- Organize outings with the team.
- Organize joint shopping expeditions.
- Eat together during lunch.
- Have a well-decorated office.
- Always encourage; do not discourage.
- Play soothing music in the work area.
- Have a clean atmosphere—protect your work area from dust and sound.
- Start a Humour Club or a Laughter Club.
- Start a book and magazine club.
- Share personal problems within the team. Respect your team members.
- To relieve stress, provide a counsellor.
- Appreciate people for their achievements.
- Share strengths and weaknesses openly.
- Celebrate birthdays and anniversaries.
- Share interesting articles.
- Share a thought for the day.
- Appreciate other people's talents.
- Do not disturb people when they are working.
- Create a friendly atmosphere.
- Make people conscious of the passage of time.
- Never use other people's possessions without telling them.
- Say hi to people and smile at them.
- Respect others.
- Establish mutual understanding.
- Help team members when they are in distress.
- Everyone should take responsibility for a job.
- Maintain open-mindness.
- Work to create meaningful personal relationships with co-workers.
- Provide time for short relaxation breaks atleast three times a day.

- Take a walk outdoors during lunch break.
- Don't get involved in politics and backbiting.
- Cultivate a hobby you love.
- If you have an unhealthy workplace look for another job.
- Celebrate achievements, even small ones.
- Make your workspace clean and comfortable. Fill it with happy pictures.

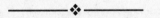

Politics in the workplace can make the blood boil with suppressed rage and unexpressed anxiety. The monsters—anger, greed and jealousy—shroud the gardens of the mind, poisoning the blood and turning the body into a desolate wasteland of disease. Today, since much of our lives are spent in the office, the corporate jungle takes an unimaginable toll on the heart. There are endless deadlines, deadly competitiveness and the need to be in a constant state of high alert. As one crisis leads to another, nature's ultimate survival mechanism of 'fight or flight' becomes a chronic response, resulting from a threat to survival. Such a response is like using an atom bomb to kill an ant.

Due to the modern urge to change jobs rapidly, many executives find themselves in threatening environments

---

Arm yourself to fight stress in the workplace

- Spend time reading and improving your mind.
- Get involved in activities that will benefit others.
- Develop an absorbing hobby.
- Get involved in the activities of your spouse and children.
- Keep in touch with close friends and extended families; use the power of the internet.
- Plan to take off from work on weekends.

- Meditate.

- Take care of yourself.

- Ponder over your goals and how your job will help you achieve them.

- Be in touch with best practices in your field.

- Learn to say 'No'.

- Network with the best professionals in your field. Meet those who love their work and enjoy it.

- People are more important than getting ahead.

- Remember that your health is more important than the car, house, bank balance or foreign holiday.

———————— ❖ ————————

surrounded by potential enemies all the time. They have no time to develop friends or trusted supporters. Everyday they walk into the modern equivalent of a jungle infested with wild animals and danger. To make it worse, family support systems are often missing. Nuclear families build up explosive pressure due to a revolution of rising expectations, fuelled by the media.

❓ Ask yourself

	Yes	No	?
Do I spend enough time reading?	☐	☐	☐
Do I effectively balance time among family, social, academic and recreational activities?	☐	☐	☐
Do I concentrate too hard on just getting the job done rather than on my whole career?	☐	☐	☐

Do I look up to my bosses as role models?	□	□	□
Do I think my bosses have double standards?	□	□	□
Do I read books, write papers and improve my knowledge to retain my job and have a good life?	□	□	□
Are there some active steps I would take today to ensure a successful future?	□	□	□
Do I talk to professionals in various fields to help improve my job awareness?	□	□	□
Is this a frightening thing to do?	□	□	□
Do I use the channels, people, or sources that could make this a pleasant experience?	□	□	□
Have I honestly assessed my potential for growth and participation in future jobs?	□	□	□
Do I travel for more than a week every month?	□	□	□
Do I rest when I am tired?	□	□	□
Have I learnt to say 'No' politely?	□	□	□
Do I set unrealistic or impossible deadlines for myself?	□	□	□
Do I take on too many jobs at once?	□	□	□
Do I eat faster than everyone else at the table?	□	□	□
Am I full of burning ambition?	□	□	□

Score

9 to 11 yeses: Good
You have found excellent balance at work. You are a joy to work with, creating positive fields for others around you. You and those who work with you will enjoy a 'heart protective environment'.

5 to 8 yeses: Adequate
You need to review some of your attitudes. The atmosphere you work in could be made more nurturing and supportive.

Less than 5 yeses: Poor
Run from this unhealthy workplace if you want to protect your heart.

○ Affirmations ○

Sit with your eyes closed and silently affirm:

- My work provides my family and me a chance to lead a comfortable life.
- I love and respect my work.
- My work provides me an opportunity to use my talents productively.
- My workplace is an opportunity to practise my skills in maintaining human relations. Conflicts are meant to be solved.
- I will not agree to do what is beyond my capacity.
- I will work sensible hours.
- I will recognize and stop stressful reactions as soon as I notice them.

- ◆ I am competent, hard-working and a good teammate.

- ◆ I will support my team and enjoy the support it gives me.

The Family

After World War II, many babies in England were orphaned. They were put in state run orphanages, kept warm and clean and fed at regular intervals. Suddenly many of the babies died of some unknown cause. Scientists believed that the reason for death was a 'lack of human touch'. These deaths were caused by lack of hugging, fondling and nurturing. No one mothered the babies or spoke to them or sang to them. The children died due to lack of love.

The family provides the love and nurturing required for the survival of children. As we grow older we crave nurturing, but are not adept at asking for it. We long for reassurance from our loved ones. We want to hear them say, 'What I really like about you is . . .' They may say it verbally, tonally or non-verbally.

The opposite of reassurance is a brush off. You need at least ten reassuring statements for every brush off to sustain a healthy relationship. A home in which no reassurances are voiced becomes a torture chamber instead of a sanctuary. Dr Dean Ornish says that men who feel that their wives love them are more likely to be capable of reversing heart disease than those who feel the opposite.

'Family is the shock absorber of society, to which the bruised and battered individual returns after doing battle with the world,' wrote Alvin Toffler in his landmark work *Future Shock*. The family provides unconditional love for the crippled, the old and the helpless. It heals the pain of failure and provides relief from the assaults of a cruel competitive world.

The home can be the cause for heart disease. It can also be the safe sanctuary for healing and reversing the heart disease. Fill your home with positive strokes and a peaceful atmosphere. Make it a nurturing space that enhances *prana* or the life force. Laughter, smiles, compliments and hugs can create a powerful positive field in the home.

 Ask yourself

	Yes	No	?
Is my family important to me?	☐	☐	☐
Do I spend adequate quality time with my family?	☐	☐	☐
Would I like to increase the amount of quality time I spend with my family?	☐	☐	☐
Does my family include those outside the nuclear family?	☐	☐	☐
Could I be a leader in making this happen?	☐	☐	☐
Is respect from my family important to me?	☐	☐	☐
Do I show appreciation for things my family has done for me?	☐	☐	☐
Do I seek to make my family life different from what I experienced while I was growing up?	☐	☐	☐

Are there things I could do to make my
family happy? ☐ ☐ ☐

Should I seek out books and classes that
would help me to be a successful parent? ☐ ☐ ☐

Does anyone in my household consume
tobacco? ☐ ☐ ☐

Does alcohol play a part in my life?
Is it a problem? ☐ ☐ ☐

Do I speak up too much or too little in
my family? ☐ ☐ ☐

Is there too much fighting in my family? ☐ ☐ ☐

Are there ways I could help reduce this? ☐ ☐ ☐

Are there too many rules in my family? ☐ ☐ ☐

Am I considerate in my handling of
misunderstandings among family members? ☐ ☐ ☐

Do I come from a broken family? ☐ ☐ ☐

Given the present situation, is there anything
I could do to strengthen my own character
or family ties? ☐ ☐ ☐

Could I possibly use outside help such as
counselling, and friends, to assist me in
attaining a solid family now or in the future? ☐ ☐ ☐

SCORE

10 to 12 yeses: Good

You are lucky to be part of a strong family unit, the most
important shield against heart disease. Celebrate it.

6 to 9 yeses: Adequate

You need to pay more attention to your family and not take these precious bonds for granted. Take out some quality time and spend a greater quantity of it with the family.

Less than 5 yeses: Poor

You must give top priority to building up your family ties. This is a must to keep your heart healthy.

○ **Affirmations** ○

Sit with your eyes closed and silently affirm:

- ◆ I have a safe and happy home.
- ◆ I enjoy unconditional love.
- ◆ The food I eat and the water I drink at home nourishes me.
- ◆ God blesses my family and keeps my children safe.
- ◆ This home is a sanctuary and a refuge.
- ◆ All conflicts in the home can be solved without anyone being hurt.

Personal

Michelangelo was once asked how he created great statues. Old and half blind, he stood before a block of marble from the quarries of Cararra, scarred and muddy. He said quietly, 'I have never created a statue. I just stand before a block of marble and study it with reverence. For I know, that within every block of marble, there lies a statue, waiting to be liberated by the touch of the Master's hand.' Similarly within each of us lies hidden a masterpiece waiting to be liberated by the magic touch of attention.

You are a powerhouse of potential. Do not allow others to influence you to think negatively about yourself by their comments. You must learn to encourage yourself and soothe yourself when you are hurt.

 Ask yourself

	Yes	No	?
Do I usually make decisions after careful thought?	☐	☐	☐
Could it be that I have allowed other people to blind me to the truth about my potential?	☐	☐	☐
Am I interested in becoming an expert on myself?	☐	☐	☐
Do I believe I can change and grow into the kind of person I really want to be?	☐	☐	☐
Do I often make emotional decisions?	☐	☐	☐
Are the results of my emotional decision-making satisfactory to me?	☐	☐	☐
Do I ever hold grudges?	☐	☐	☐
Are the people that I hold grudges against members of my own family?	☐	☐	☐
Would I feel better if I refused to hold grudges and instead cleared the air when problems arose?	☐	☐	☐

Do I handle my emotions in a mature way? □ □ □

Could I improve the way I handle my emotions? □ □ □

Do I know anyone with whom I can confidently
share my emotions? □ □ □

Do I have some activities that help me
release pressure and tension? □ □ □

Do I generally accept my feelings as
being an important part of me? □ □ □

Do I have any habits that get in my way and
keep me from growing and changing? □ □ □

Do I like the picture that I hold of myself as I
interact with others? □ □ □

Do I like the picture of myself as I relate
to others? □ □ □

Do I have pictures of myself that I might
like to change? □ □ □

Are my goals clear to me? □ □ □

Do I often replay in my mind the negative
experiences of the past? □ □ □

Is it easy for me to understand new concepts
or ideas? □ □ □

Am I good at creatively finding solutions
to problems? □ □ □

Do I ever try to visualize the outcome of
events before they happen? □ □ □

Am I satisfied with my attitude towards work? □ □ □

Have I ever given serious consideration to
my attitudes? □ □ □

Am I aware of attitudes I have that are
blocking my growth? □ □ □

Do the opinions of others influence my
attitude towards other people? □ □ □

Do I want to make my own decisions and
generate my own attitudes? □ □ □

Am I aware that other people and the media
are always trying to condition me to
think the way they do? Am I aware of
hidden persuaders? □ □ □

Do I carefully select the people I allow
to condition me? □ □ □

Do I carefully select my music, books,
movies, etc.? □ □ □

Am I a positive conditioner of the people
around me? □ □ □

Is it possible for me to determine how
others see me? □ □ □

Am I missing opportunities because of
my conditioning? □ □ □

Do I allow others to condition me by
letting them be an expert on me? □ □ □

Would I like to be an expert on myself? □ □ □

Are my goals clear to me? □ □ □

Am I actively seeking information to help
me achieve my goals? □ □ □

Are the pictures I hold of my goals positive? □ □ □

Do I often limit my seeking of goals because
I can't see exactly how I could ever
achieve them? □ □ □

Do I limit myself by what I believe is
possible or impossible? □ □ □

Do I have confidence and faith in my ability
to accomplish goals? □ □ □

Would I like to be more confident? □ □ □

Do I admire people around me who always
seem to be winning or achieving? □ □ □

Do I know how to make myself comfortable
in uncomfortable situations? □ □ □

Have my feelings of stress and tension ever
kept me from doing as well as I know I can? □ □ □

Do I often feel nervous or tense when I am
around new or different people? □ □ □

Would I be nervous interviewing for a job
or a contract? □ □ □

Do my emotions keep me from taking
tests successfully ? □ □ □

Would I perform up to my ability
even under stressful situations? □ □ □

Do I ever stop and listen to what I say to
myself about my past performance? ☐ ☐ ☐

Do my past performances affect today's
performances? ☐ ☐ ☐

Will today's performance influence
tomorrow's or next year's performances? ☐ ☐ ☐

Score

Between 37 and 28 yeses: Good
You have a positive, winning attitude and people like being
around you. You are an achiever.

27 and 15 yeses: Adequate
You sometimes allow yourself to succumb to negative
thoughts. Stop internalizing destructive criticism. Get out
of your comfort zone and start encouraging yourself.

Less than 14 yeses: Poor
You allow others to define you negatively. Seek out a close
friend or a counsellor to help you.

○ Affirmations ○

Sit with your eyes closed and silently affirm:

- By nature I am kind, gentle and loving.
- Any mistake I have committed is unintentional and
  I forgive myself for it.

- God's grace has created a magic circle of love, a safety net for my loved ones and me.
- I am capable of achieving my goals with hard work and dedication.
- I will look around me for help and knowledge to reach my goals.
- I will seek companions who will encourage and help me.
- God is with me.

Ethics and Morals

It has been proved by studies conducted in the Harvard School of Medicine that altruistic, volunteer work increases the body's capacity to fight disease and remain healthy. Being kind is certainly the path towards good health. Perhaps the ancient Hindu belief that all souls are part of the divine being and are therefore connected ensures that when we make others happy, we receive a jolt of bliss ourselves. When we make others sad, we receive a dose of health-destroying poison.

When we are aware that we may not be living up to our own standards, the body punishes us with a feeling of unease. The symptoms of restlessness, insomnia and raised blood pressure are the inevitable results.

Dharma or right action, bestows the gift of a quiet mind. *Dharma* is the ancient Indian golden rule of righteousness. This includes being truthful, doing your duty without worrying about the results, treating all forms of life with reverence, non-violence and peace. When a man lives by his *dharma*, he inherits health and peace, because he lives in harmony with the laws of the land and the laws of God. 'The wages of sin are death,' says the Bible. The wages of sin are certainly illness as tension and anxiety create the unease and toxins and diseases flourish in the body. A peaceful, noble heart is a healthy heart.

❓ Ask yourself

	Yes	No	?
Do I ever hold myself responsible for the ethics or moral standards of others?	☐	☐	☐
Do I feel any responsibility for the poor, crippled or sick?	☐	☐	☐
Are my ethical standards based on what others have told me in the past?	☐	☐	☐
Have I made my own decisions about what is honest and right?	☐	☐	☐
Are honesty and integrity important to me?	☐	☐	☐
Do I ever rationalize (make excuses)?	☐	☐	☐
Do I have a role in seeing that others are protected against unfairness or injustice?	☐	☐	☐
Am I as concerned with the quality of life of others as I am with the quality of my own family's life?	☐	☐	☐
Is the golden rule 'treat others as you want to be treated yourself' a principle I live by?	☐	☐	☐

Score

7 to 5 yeses: Good
You do what you say and think, whether others are watching or not. Results: good sleep and a healthy appetite.

4 to 3 yeses: Adequate
Some double standards cause you concern in your subconscious. Get rid of them. A little more compassion in your treatment of others may help.

Less than 3 yeses: Poor
Review and make drastic changes in the double life you are leading. It places terrible stress on the heart.

○ Affirmations ○

Sit with your eyes closed and affirm silently:

- ◆ I will live by my own moral standards.
- ◆ I do what I preach.
- ◆ I will help all and harm no one.
- ◆ Peace and goodwill surround me at all times.

Chapter 7

HEAL YOUR HEART NATURALLY

Absorb the sun's energy

The sun is the source of all life. Choose a time when the sun is not too hot—before 8 a.m. in the morning or after 6.00 p.m. Wear comfortable clothes and sit on a thick mat or *dhurrie* in a place that you consider special.

Close your eyes and be still. Breathe gently and attune yourself to the rhythm of your breathing. Imagine the sunlight entering your body and filling every part of your body with energy.

Chant the holy 'Om' as you breathe in. With your hand on your navel, breathe in the energy of the sun. As you breathe out, feel all the impure and stale, toxic waste leaving your body.

Imagine the brilliance of the sun in your face. Imagine the might of the sun touching and healing and energizing your family, your friends and the whole earth. Everywhere you look, everything you touch will be energized by the sun.

The *Gayathri Mantra* which seeks to infuse the body with the energy of the sun has been used by Indians for thousands of years to instil the sun's energy in the body, mind and spirit. Learn the mantra from a guru or teacher.

Meditate

Sit calmly in a quiet and tranquil spot. The spot should get a lot of air and sunlight. Breathe peacefully and deeply. Let your mind be calm. When you breathe in, take in all the energies of the universe. When you breathe out, exhale all the toxins, anxiety and pain from your body. If thoughts interfere, let them pass by like clouds in the sky.

Enjoy the silence. Carry this silence into the noise and haste of the world around you. Your restful presence will soothe all those among you.

Close your eyes and place your feet flat on the ground. Make sure your spine is erect and your breathing is slow and even. Visualize your heart in the centre of your chest, towards the left side. Place your left hand over your heart and then place the right hand over it.

Breathe in and out gently, concentrating on your breath. Pay attention to each part of your body and consciously relax your body from the tips of your toes to the top of your head.

The Bhagavad Gita says

On a clean spot, which is neither too high nor too low, a seat should be made with Kusa grass, with a cloth spread over it. Firmly seated on it, the Yogi should practise spiritual communion, with mind concentrated and with the working of the imaginative faculty and the senses under control, for self-purification.

The flame of a lamp sheltered from wind does not flicker. This is the comparison used to describe a Yogi's mind that is well under control and united with the Atman.

Affirm to yourself

- My heart is becoming stronger, kinder and healthier with every passing day.
- With every passing day my arteries are becoming clean and flexible.
- Everyday my heart beats regularly and strongly.
- My heart will be healed by the grace of god.
- As you continue to breathe in and out, repeat ten times each: 'Om', 'Oo', 'Ah'.

Laugh

In his book *Humour and Ageing* psychiatrist William Fry writes that it is estimated that the impact on the heart of twenty seconds of hearty laughter is comparable to three minutes of rowing, which is supposed to be the best aerobic exercise for reconditioning the entire body and promoting longevity. He goes on to say that laughter stimulates the heart, supplies oxygen to the lungs and energizes the brain cells, which promotes a positive outlook in life.

Laughter introduces chemicals of happiness into the bloodstream and reduces pain in every part of the body. It is essential in the process of reversal of heart disease. You should learn to relax and break into a smile as often as possible. Always remember that it takes just twenty-six muscles to smile while all of sixty-two muscles are used while frowning.

Spiritual Healing

Sri Aurobindo writes about a spiritual concept of health: 'For nearly forty years I believed them when they said I was weakly in constitution, suffered constantly from the smaller and greater ailments and mistook this curse for a burden that Nature had laid upon me. When I renounced the aid of medicines, then they began to depart from me like disappointed parasites. Then only I understood what a mighty force was the natural health within me and how much mightier yet the Will and Faith exceeding mind which God meant to be the divine support of our life in this body . . .'

An integral view of health demands an integral view of life. To attune the different elements of our nature to this view of life as the central nucleus is the next step. Without such reorientation and reorganization it will not be possible to establish in ourselves the law of harmony and peace which is so necessary a condition for integral health.

'It is true that human impatience readily rushes to all that appears to it instantaneous and miraculous . . . To conquer our inner nature and resolve the conflict ridden, divided existence that we lead, into a harmonious integrated whole is necessary for a healthy and wholesome living,' said Vijay Poddar, in NAMAHA (New Approaches to Medicine and Health).

Our personal healthcare systems are determined by the traditional habits, lifestyle and value systems of the particular culture from where it has evolved. They cannot be effective if there is a radical change in the habits of that culture. This 'patient-system mismatch' is very evident in the case of Red Indians who have lost their traditional healing capacities. On the contrary, people from Kerala, in spite of coming into contact with Western culture, still value their traditions. Perhaps that is why their age-old high-cholesterol diet has not resulted in an increased incidence of heart disease.

Yoga

The word 'yoga' is derived from the sanskrit word 'yuj' which means 'to yoke, attach or join'.

Yoga is one of the six *darshanas*: it provides a mirror in which we may see ourselves and realize our full potential. Yoga tries to condition the body and the mind so that we are always present in every action at every moment. It is the ultimate mindfulness that helps us to dive into every moment and experience it fully. It helps us become full participants in life instead of distracted spectators. The classic definition of yoga is, of course, 'to be one with the Lord'.

The science of yoga was systematized by Maharishi Patanjanli into 285 *yogasutras*. According to Patanjali's *yogasutras*, the senses are the doors of perception. There are nine types of interruption in the individual's journey to the state of yoga and union with the divine. They are illness, mental stagnation, doubt, lack of foresight, fatigue, overindulgence, illusions about one's true state of mind, lack of perseverance and regression.

Patanjali lays down eight steps to achieve union with the Lord:

Yama: Universal moral commandments.

Niyama: Self-purification by discipline.

Asana: Posture.

Pranayama: Rhythmic control of breath.

Pratyahara: Withdrawal of the mind from the domination of the senses and exterior objects.

Dharna: Concentration.

Dhyana: Meditation.

Samadhi: Thoughtless state in which one becomes one unites with the object of his meditation.

Here we shall deal with the third stage, namely the asanas. Yogasana combines effortless postures and definite stances in the projection of a healthy and striking personality. It involves the harmony of bodily stances and breathing techniques that mould every part of the body to its ideal contour. This is possible through various postures or asanas which also enhance one's personality. Asanas are thus not merely yogic postures, they embody the proper physical and mental disposition through the harmony of body and mind.

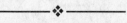

Before you begin the asanas

☐ The qualities needed in yoga students are: discipline and perseverance to practice regularly without interruption.

☐ Before doing asanas your bladder and bowels should be emptied.

☐ Asanas are to be done on an empty stomach. You may have one cup of milk or coffee fifteen minutes before. Allow at least four hours to elapse after a heavy meal. Food may be eaten thirty minutes after completing asanas.

☐ Choose any place free from insects and noise. Do not perform asanas on the bare floor, but on a folded blanket on a levelled floor.

☐ Stay in each yogic posture as long as you can.

☐ Deep breathing in every posture is essential.

☐ Always perform asanas on both sides, namely left and right, for equal durations of time.

Yogasadhana for heart ailments

The following asanas are simple and known to be effective in ensuring a healthy heart. They should be learnt from a competent guru or an instructor.

PADMASANA

Padmasana brings harmony between the body, mind and soul. Those who suffer from anxiety, tension or anger can practise this asana to experience peace of mind.

This asana also cures heart and lung diseases and digestive disorders, as well as sciatica and rheumatism of the legs.

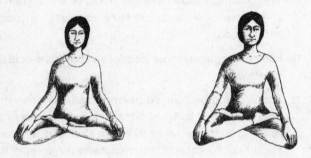

DHANURASANA

Dhanurasana is an excellent asana for the spinal cord. It strengthens the hips and takes care of spondylitis. It expands the chest and increases blood circulation in the heart muscles.

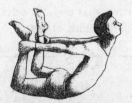

SARVANGASANA

This asana expands the ribcage and helps in deep breathing. It also increases the lung capacity. The inverted body pose brings fresh supply of oxygen-rich blood to the heart. It counteracts fatigue and exhaustion. Note: This asana should not be done by those with heart disease.

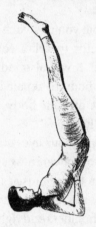

MATSYASANA

This asana expands your chest and tones the nerves of the neck and back. It is very beneficial for those suffering from bronchial congestion, asthma and other respiratory diseases. It also ensures that the thyroid and parathyroid glands obtain maximum benefit.

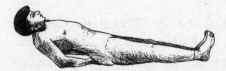

SAVASANA

Savasana helps the body to relax totally, almost like a corpse. People who are tense and disturbed can benefit from this asana because it pacifies the mind and rejuvenates the body.

YOGA NIDRA

Yoga nidra will enable you to switch off from your everyday life and relax. It helps to relax your tense muscles even while you are awake. It will also induce a deep sleep which is necessary for the body to repair and renew itself. Learn to talk to each part of your body as you breathe gently, evenly and peacefully.

As you breathe with your eyes shut talk to every muscle of your body. Shift your awareness slowly from the muscles of your toes, right up to the muscles of your head and face, and ensure that they are relaxed. Pay particular attention to the muscles of your shoulders and right arm which are usually more tense than the rest of the body. Soothe and relax the muscles of your jaws and forehead and back of the neck. The muscles of the stomach are usually scrunched with tension and require special attention.

When you breathe in, feel your whole body fill with oxygen and the powerful energies of the universe. When you breathe out, let every bit of tension and stale air leave your body.

PRANAYAMA

Pranayama, the art of regulating and controlling your breathing, is distinct from deep breathing which is merely inhalation and exhalation of air. Pranayama involves voluntarily changing the rhythms of intake and outflow of air into the lungs, using its full capacity, and holding the breath for a fixed period of time following a particular rhythm.

Apart from calming the mind and improving metabolism, pranayama increases the body's resistance against respiratory diseases.

Does yoga work?

Although yoga is not a system of medicine, adoption of some selected elements of the yogic lifestyle for relatively short periods of time, even half-heartedly, seems to have favourable effects on health. Physiological effects of some yogic practices are well documented.

Research in this field has revealed the following facts:

- Dr B.K.Anand and his colleagues at the All India Institute of Medical Sciences (AIIMS) made some classic observations, which were published in 1961. First, they observed a preponderance of alpha activity (during which the brain produces waves that keep the mind relaxed but alert) in the EEG of yogis. Further, sensory stimuli such as a loud bang or ice-cold water which normally block the alpha rhythm, could not do so in yogis while they were meditating.

- Wallace demonstrated a reduction in oxygen consumption as well as heart rate during transcendental meditation.

- Recent studies have explored some finer effects of yogic practices. For example, it was observed that during 'om' meditation there was a significant reduction in heart rate but an increase in cuteaneous peripheral vascular resistance, indicating a physiologically relaxed state but increased mental alertness.

- A significant fall in systolic as well as diastolic blood pressure followed meditation in twenty-two borderline hypertensive patients.

- In another study, transcendental meditation for twelve weeks led to a transient but significant fall in blood pressure in six out of seven hypertensive patients. However, the fall in anxiety scores was both significant and sustained.

- It has also been reported that yogic practices tilt the autonomic function towards parasympathetic dominance. Although the parasympathetic activity becomes relatively more, there is also an increase in adrenocortical secretion, or the secretion of adrenaline by the adrenal glands in some situations, which has been hypothesized to improve the organism's ability to cope with stress. This may be expected to have a protective or calming effect on the heart, blood vessels, gastrointestinal system and several other organs.

Muscle relaxation and other techniques

Just as you tighten your right hand into a fist and then totally relax it, try to tighten groups of muscles in your body and relax them. This will teach you how a tight muscle feels as opposed to a relaxed one. You will then become aware of the difference between tension and relaxation. Progressive muscle relaxation is a well-known technique that was developed by Edmund Jacobson in 1930. The Lamaze technique which is practised to ensure easy childbirth is also useful in promoting muscle relaxation. Self-hypnosis can help you enhance the force of positive suggestions and affirmations to learn good habits. Pranic healing and therapeutic massage are part of the process of healing and may be used after learning the proper techniques from well-known practitioners.

————— ❖ —————

Integrate exercise into your daily routine

☐ Work in the garden and with plants.

☐ Keep a pet.

☐ Walk up steps.

☐ Walk around your home, look under beds.

☐ Cycle on a stationary bike as you watch TV.

☐ Walk down to the vegetable shop.

☐ Walk to the coffee shop or machine.

————— ❖ —————

Shiatsu and Reflexology

Shiatsu is a form of therapy of Japanese origin based on the principles of acupuncture. It involves the application of pressure on certain points on the body using the hands.

Tension in the hands, wrist and forearm is common for many of us who are constantly working on the computer. You can help yourself with the following exercise.

Grasp your left hand with your right. Using your thumb and forefinger, touch the 108 energy points on the hand. Put pressure on the point between the thumb and first finger and hold it for five seconds.

Reflexology is a similar technique used on the energy points on the feet. Use your hands and press from the base of the big toe to the heel. Pay special attention to the Achilles tendon. A foot massage or even a pedicure is one of the most effective methods of inducing relaxation and relieving yourself of tension.

Chapter 8

THE ZERO HEART ATTACK DIET

The ZHAP diet is a low-fat diet plan aimed at lowering your cholesterol levels and reducing the risk of suffering from a heart ailment. Normally 'healthy' diets are believed to comprise salads, soups and boiled vegetables, which most people find unpalatable. The resulting inability to stick to the regimen often causes anxiety and depression in the individual.

---❖---

Preparing to eat a healthy meal

- Prepare to eat, by being silent to calm the body.
- Breathe peacefully from the naval for a few minutes.
- Eat in silence.
- If you must speak while you eat, talk about happy events and subjects.
- Do not eat with someone who irritates you or makes you angry.
- Make sure you eat in good company.
- Switch off the TV and the computer while you are eating.
- Ignore phones and pagers.
- Listen to soothing music or mantras.
- Do not eat when you are angry or distressed. Drink cold water or fresh juice and wait till you are calm. Eat atleast six small meals a day.

---❖---

The ZHAP diet is a new, specially designed, low-fat diet plan which tastes as good as your normal food and which you will be able to adhere to without much difficulty. It is low in substances that are bad for your health and rich in substances that will protect you against heart disease and other illnesses. These meals are not meant just for the person at risk; they are for the whole family. This has two obvious benefits: one, you need not cook two sets of meals; two, the person at risk is not tempted by the food consumed by others.

Salient features of the ZHAP diet

This is a purely vegetarian diet which includes vegetables, fruits, pulses, grains and non-fat dairy products. It excludes all kinds of oils, butter, ghee, cheese, processed foods and coconut. Of course, it goes without saying that sweets, fried items and alcohol are not a part of it.

Contrary to what is usually believed, there is no significant loss of taste due to the lack of oils, coconut and butter. Seasoning of curries, dals and sambars is more a matter of habit and dispensing with it doesn't really affect the taste of the particular dish. Coconuts can be substituted in some dishes with different dals which have a similar texture and taste. Use of butter in soups can be avoided by pureeing the cooked vegetables and adding a little bit of skimmed milk. In salads, try to use low-fat yoghurt, lemon juice and vinegar instead of salad oil. Breakfast items like dosas should be prepared in a non-stick pan, which requires very small quantities of oil. It is perfectly possible to make common food items taste good without too much of fat content. By following such general principles, you can suitably modify your own favourite recipes into low-fat items.

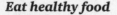The ZHAP diet involves a thirty-day low-fat diet plan, which you should adopt in a cycle for the next six months. The diet plan includes six items for breakfast, six varieties of soups, twelve salads and twenty-six main dishes for lunch and dinner. In addition, consumption of at least eight to ten glasses of water is essential daily.

Eat healthy food

- Be careful what you put into your mouth. Make sure everything you eat is fresh, clean and full of *prana*.

- Do not eat processed or frozen food as far as possible.

- Drink at least eight glasses of water every day.

- The Indian diet has a lot of carbohydrates and whole grains, dals, legumes, fresh vegetables and fruits. Carbohydrates found in whole grains stimulate the production of 'the happiness chemical', seretonium. They also provide Vitamin B and pantothermic acid which fight the lethal stress chemicals.

- Water is a great cleanser. It helps the body wash out toxins and the lethal chemicals of stress. Unless the doctor forbids it, drink eight glasses of warm water every day.

- Avoid stimulants like coffee, aerated drinks and cigarettes. Light herbal teas are a great replacement.

- Reduce the intake of salt—your body needs only one-fifth the amount of salt usually used in Indian food.

- Reduce intake of ghee and all oils as much as possible. You are probably consuming nine times the oil you need if you eat a normal Indian diet. High levels of cholesterol with the precarious genetic heritage of thinner arteries in Indians is a lethal combination.

- Eat generous amounts of fibre, fresh fruits and vegetables.

THE ZHAP DIET PLAN

BREAKFAST DISHES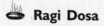

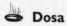 ### Ragi Dosa

½ cup urad dal

¼ cup rice

3 cups ragi flour

Salt to taste

Soak the rice and dal for three to four hours, and then grind to a smooth paste. To the ground mixture add the ragi flour along with salt and enough water to form a smooth, firm paste. Leave overnight to ferment. Make the dosa on a non-stick tava.

You can add chopped onions, curry leaves, coriander and green chillies to the batter before making the dosa.

Dosa

2 cups rice

¼ cup urad dal

¼ cup boiled rice

1 tsp tur dal

½ tsp fenugreek seeds

Salt to taste

Soak the dals and rice and fenugreek seeds for three to four hours. Grind to a smooth paste. Add salt and ferment overnight.

Make the dosas the next morning on a non-stick tava without any oil.

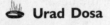

Oothappam

To the normal dosa batter add:

Chopped onions

Green chillies

Coriander leaves

¼ tsp turmeric

A few curry leaves

Mix the ingredients well and make the oothappam the next day.

Urad Dosa

2 cups rice

½ cup urad dal

Salt to taste

Soak dal and rice for three to four hours. Grind to a smooth paste. Add salt and ferment overnight. Make thick dosas the next day.

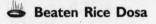 **Beaten Rice Dosa**

3 cups rice (soak for three to four hours)

I cup beaten rice (awal)

I cup curd

Salt to taste

Grind the rice, beaten rice and curd to a paste. Add salt and ferment overnight. Make dosas with the fermented mixture next morning.

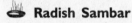 **Radish Sambar**

½ cup tur dal

3-4 white radish, chopped in medium pieces

2 tomatoes, chopped

I onion, chopped

Tamarind (small bits)

Salt to taste

To be ground after roasting:

3-4 dry red chillies

½ tsp jeera

¼ tsp fenugreek seeds

2 tsp coriander seeds

I tsp channa dal

2 tsp urad dal

¼ tsp turmeric powder

A pinch of hing

Add the tamarind to the roasted ingredients and grind to a coarse paste. To the cooked dal add chopped radish, salt and the ground masala. Let it boil till the radish is cooked well.

Pressure cook the dal with the tomatoes and onion.

Soups

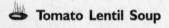 Palak Soup

1 big bunch of palak leaves

½ cup milk (cold)

1 tsp cornflour

Salt and pepper to taste

Boil the palak with a little salt. Purée it in a blender. Pour the purée into a pan and let it boil. While it is boiling, add the milk after mixing cornflour with it. Let it boil for five to seven minutes. Add pepper and salt. Remove when the consistency is slightly thick and serve.

Tomato Lentil Soup

½ cup split yellow dal (moong)

4 big tomatoes, peeled

1 onion, chopped

1 small carrot, grated

1 tsp chilli powder

¼ tsp jeera powder

1 tsp lemon powder

1 tsp lemon juice

Chopped coriander leaves

Salt to taste

Put the dal, tomatoes and onion in a cooker along with four glasses of water and pressure cook for ten to fifteen minutes. Mash the oiled vegetables well with a spoon. Add the masala powders and grated carrot and let it boil for seven to eight minutes. Remove from fire and add lemon juice. Before serving, garnish with grated carrot and coriander leaves.

Mixed Vegetable Soup

1 carrot, grated

6 beans, chopped

¼ cup chopped cabbage

½ bunch spinach

1 onion, quartered

1 tomato, chopped

½ cup milk (cold)

1 tsp cornflour

Salt and pepper to taste

Put all the vegetables, the onion and the tomato in a cooker along with two big glasses of water, and pressure cook for fifteen minutes. When cooked, strain the vegetables and blend them in a mixie. Mix the blended vegetables to the previously strained water and boil, adding more water if necessary. When it starts to boil, add salt, pepper and milk to which cornflour is added. Let it boil for five minutes.

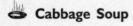 Cabbage Soup

I cup chopped cabbage

I carrot, chopped

I medium potato, chopped

I onion

¼ cup milk

Salt and pepper to taste

Pressure cook the cabbage, carrot, potato and onion along with three cups of water.

Strain and purée it. Mix the purée with the strained water and boil in the milk for three to four minutes. Add salt and pepper to taste.

Cauliflower Soup

2 cups cauliflower florets (soaked in hot salted water for a few minutes)

I onion, chopped

3 cups water

Salt and pepper to taste

Coriander leaves (for garnishing)

Pressure cook the cauliflower, onion and water for twelve to fifteen minutes. Make a purée and bring to a boil. Season with salt and pepper. Before serving garnish with coriander leaves.

Palak-Mushroom Soup

1 cup palak, chopped (50 g)

1 cup mushroom, sliced (70 g)

4 bulbs spring onion, chopped

½ cup milk

Salt and pepper to taste

Put the palak, mushroom, onions and salt in a cooker, and sauté for three to four minutes. Add two cups of water and pressure cook for ten minutes. When it cools, make a purée and bring to a boil. Add milk and pepper. Let it boil for a few minutes.

MAIN MEALS

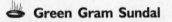 Green Gram Sundal

1 cup green gram

1 onion

1-2 green chillies

¼ tsp mustard

½ tsp urad dal

A few curry leaves

1 tsp lemon juice

Salt to taste

Cook the green gram in a pressure cooker for about eight to ten minutes. Add all the other ingredients to the cooked gram and leave it on a low flame for a few minutes until dry.

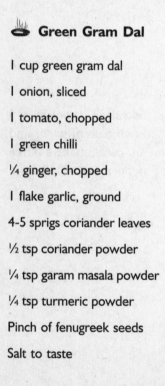 **Green Gram Dal**

1 cup green gram dal

1 onion, sliced

1 tomato, chopped

1 green chilli

¼ ginger, chopped

1 flake garlic, ground

4-5 sprigs coriander leaves

½ tsp coriander powder

¼ tsp garam masala powder

¼ tsp turmeric powder

Pinch of fenugreek seeds

Salt to taste

Put all the ingredients in a cooker except the coriander and garam masala powder. Add enough water (four to five glasses) and pressure cook for about half an hour. When it is well cooked, mash with a spoon and add the masala powders and let it boil for a few minutes.

Tur Dal

½ cup tur dal

I onion, sliced

I tomato, chopped

I green chilli

½ tsp ginger, pounded

2-3 sprigs coriander leaves

¼ tsp turmeric powder

Salt to taste

Put all the ingredients except the coriander leaves in a cooker along with two to three glasses of water. Pressure cook for fifteen minutes. When well cooked, mash the dal with a spoon. Garnish with coriander leaves before serving.

Methi Dal

½ cup tur dal

I onion, chopped

I tomato, chopped

2-3 sprigs coriander leaves

1 bunch methi leaves (fenugreek)

1-2 flakes garlic, chopped

1-2 tsp sambar powder

1 tsp lemon juice

¼ tsp turmeric powder

Salt to taste

Pinch of hing

Pressure cook the dal with turmeric powder, onion and tomato. Beat well. Add the other ingredients (except lemon juice) and pressure cook for another five to seven minutes. Mix well. Add lemon juice and let it boil for four to five minutes.

Black Dal

½ cup black urad dal

1 onion, sliced

2 tomatoes, sliced

2-3 green chillies

3-4 flakes garlic, pounded

¼ tsp turmeric powder

Salt to taste

Soak the dal for three to four hours. Pressure cook all the ingredients until they are well cooked. Beat well and let it boil for a few minutes. Garnish with coriander leaves.

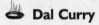 **Dal Curry**

½ cup tur dal (120 g)

½ tsp turmeric powder

½ tsp jaggery

1 tsp tamarind pulp

Coriander leaves

1 green chilli, slit

A pinch of hing

Salt to taste

To be roasted dry and then powdered:

½ tsp coriander seeds

½ tsp fenugreek seeds

1 tsp jeera

1 tsp urad dal

Pressure cook the dal with turmeric powder and about four cups of water. Stir well. Add the other ingredients along with salt and boil for about fifteen minutes. Garnish with coriander leaves.

Mixed Dal Curry

¼ cup tur dal (40 g)

¼ cup split yellow dal

¼ cup urad dal (27.5 g)

½ tsp ginger, chopped

½ tsp sugar

½ tsp garam masala

½ tsp turmeric powder

3-4 green chillies, slit

2 tomatoes, chopped

2 drumsticks, cut into medium pieces

2 brinjals, cut into cubes

Pinch of hing

Salt to taste

Soak the dals for one hour. Pressure cook with tomatoes, turmeric powder, ginger and green chillies. Beat well. Add salt and the other ingredients, and cook again until the vegetables are tender.

Dal with Spinach Curry

½ cup tur dal

1 big bunch of spinach

2 tomatoes, chopped

1 onion, quartered

2-3 flakes of garlic, ground

1½ -2 tsp sambar powder

¼ tsp turmeric powder

Pinch of hing

Salt to taste

Pressure cook the dal, onion, tomato and turmeric for about ten minutes. Then add the spinach, garlic, hing, salt and sambar powder, and pressure cook again for five to six minutes. Allow it to cool. Strain, and keep the water separately. Blend the dal and the green mixture for a few seconds (coarsely), add the strained water, and boil for a while.

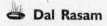 Simple Tomato Rasam

4-5 big, ripe tomatoes, mashed

4-5 sprigs coriander leaves

A few curry leaves

¼ tsp mustard seeds

Salt to taste

To be coarsely ground:

1 tsp jeera

½ tsp pepper

3-4 flakes garlic

Heat a pan, add the curry leaves and the powdered masala and stir for two minutes. Then add the well mashed tomatoes and salt. Cover and cook for eight to ten minutes. Add two to three glasses of water. Let it boil for another ten minutes. Garnish with coriander leaves and serve.

Dal Rasam

3 tbsp split yellow dal (moong)

2 tomatoes, quartered

1 tsp mustard seeds

¼ tsp turmeric

½ tsp jaggery

1 tsp oil

Curry leaves

2-3 red chillies

Salt to taste

To be pounded coarsely:

1 tsp jeera

½ tsp peppercorns

4-5 flakes garlic

Pressure cook the dal, tomato, turmeric and salt with two glasses of water. When cooked, mash well.

Heat oil and add mustard, red chillies and curry leaves. Add the pounded masala and stir for a minute. Pour the dal into this. Add jaggery and a glass of water, and let it boil for a few minutes. Garnish with coriander leaves.

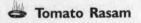 ## Tomato Rasam

2 big tomatoes

3-4 sprigs coriander leaves

½ lime-sized tamarind

A few curry leaves

To be pounded coarsely:

1 tsp jeera

1 tsp pepper corns

3-4 flakes garlic

Mash the tomatoes well and add all the other ingredients including salt. Add three to four cups of water, and mix well. Bring to a boil and when it foams remove from the fire. Cover and let it stand for a while before serving.

Vegetable Saag

2 cups mixed vegetables (beans, carrots, peas, cauliflower, etc.)

2 medium onions, sliced

4-5 green chillies, chopped

½ tsp jeera

2 tbsp roasted bengal gram

5-6 sprigs coriander leaves

¼ ginger, chopped

¼ tsp turmeric powder

2 tomatoes, chopped

2 tbsp curd

Salt to taste

Heat the pan and stir the onions and green chillies in a little bit of water in the pan. When the onions become transparent add the jeera, gram, ginger and coriander leaves, and fry for two minutes. Add turmeric powder and grind all the ingredients into to a coarse paste.

Boil the vegetables with salt and one glass of water. Add the ground masala and cook a while. Finally add the curd and tomato and cook for another eight to ten minutes till the gravy thickens.

Capsicum Kurma

3 capsicums cut in long slices

1 onion, sliced

1 tbsp coriander seeds

¼ ginger, chopped

2 cloves

½ cinnamon

1 tbsp til

¼ tsp turmeric powder

1 tsp khus khus

3 red chillies

3-4 garlic flakes

1 tsp channa dal

1 tsp urad dal

A bit of tamarind

Dry roast the coriander seeds, khus khus, til, urad and channa dals. Add the red chillies and spices and fry for a minute. Remove and add ginger, garlic and tamarind. Grind everything together to form a paste.

Heat a pan and stir the onion and capsica for five minutes, in little water.

Add the masala, salt and one cup of water. Let it cook till dry.

Vegetable Kurma

2 cups mixed vegetables (peas, carrots, beans, potatoes, cauliflower)

2 tomatoes

2 sprigs pudina leaves

5-6 sprigs coriander leaves

2 tsp water

Grind to a paste:

4 green chillies

1 onion

¼ tsp saunf

¼ tsp ginger

4 flakes garlic

1 tsp khus khus

4 cloves

½ cinnamon

2 cardamom

1 tsp oil

Heat a non-stick pan and stir the pudina and coriander in water. Add the ground masala and tomato, and mix well.

Then add the vegetables, salt and enough water to cook the vegetables. When the vegetables are cooked and the gravy is thick, remove from fire and garnish with coriander leaves.

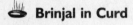 **Brinjal in Curd**

2 big brinjals

½ cup curd

¼ tsp garlic paste

1-2 green chillies

4-5 sprigs coriander leaves

Salt to taste

Roast the brinjals directly on the gas flame until it is sufficiently brown. Place in a bowl of cold water, peel off the outer cover and deseed. Keep the pulp separately.

Beat the curd well and add garlic. Mix well and keep in the fridge for about half an hour. Remove and add chopped green chillies, coriander leaves and the brinjal pulp along with salt. Mix well and serve.

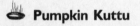 **Pumpkin Kuttu**

1 cup white pumpkin pieces

¼ cup split moong dal

1 tomato, chopped

Salt to taste

To be ground after roasting:

½ tsp jeera

1 green chilli

2 pieces each of cinnamon and cloves

1 tsp khus khus

¼ tsp turmeric

1 tbsp channa dal

1 tbsp urad dal

Boil water and add the dal to it. While it is getting cooked add the pumpkin and let it cook for a few more minutes. Then add the chopped tomato, salt and the ground masala. Let it boil for eight to ten minutes, until the gravy thickens.

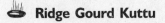 **Ridge Gourd Kuttu**

2 medium size ridge gourds

1/3 cup channa dal

1 tomato

To be ground to a paste:

3-4 dry red chillies

1 tbsp coriander seeds

1 tbsp khus khus

1 onion

¼ cinnamon

3-4 cloves

4-5 sprigs coriander leaves

¼ tsp turmeric

In a cooker put together the dal and tomato, and pressure cook for ten minutes. To this add the gourd, ground masala and salt, and let it boil on a slow flame for about fifteen minutes. You can add a few drops of lemon juice before serving.

🍲 Dry Masala Vegetables

1 cup mixed vegetables (beans, carrot, peas, cauliflower, etc.)

1 onion

3-4 sprigs coriander leaves

½ tsp jeera powder

¼ tsp red chilli powder

¼ tsp turmeric

Salt to taste

To be ground to a paste:

1 tsp channa dal

1 tsp urad dal (roasted till golden)

¼ tsp ginger

2-3 cloves garlic

In a pan, put together all the above-mentioned ingredients along with one and a half cups of water. Cover and cook until vegetables are tender. Boil till dry.

Spinach and Karamani Poriyal

1 bunch spinach

½ cup karamani (black-eyed beans)

1 onion

1-2 green chillies, slit

2-3 sprigs coriander leaves

1 tsp lemon juice

Salt to taste

Cook the karamani until it is almost done. Add the chopped spinach, onion, green chillies, coriander leaves and salt. Continue to cook. When well cooked and almost dry, add lemon juice and take it off the flame.

Potato Fry

2 big potatoes, peeled and cubed

2 big onions, quartered

1 big tomato, sliced

1 tsp sambar powder

¼ tsp jeera powder

1 tsp lemon juice

1 tbsp coriander leaves

In a non-stick pan put the potatoes, tomato, onions, sambar powder, jeera powder and salt. Add a cup of water. Cover and cook on a low flame until the potatoes are tender. Open the lid, add the coriander leaves and lemon juice and fry until dry.

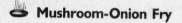

Mushroom-Onion Fry

4 cups mushroom, sliced (280 g)

2 cups onions, sliced

½ tsp pepper powder

Salt to taste

Put the mushrooms and onions in a non-stick pan with a little salt and sprinkle a little water. Sauté without covering for three to four minutes. Cover and cook for five to seven minutes. If it becomes too dry, sprinkle a little water now and then. Open the lid, add the pepper and continue to fry for a few minutes.

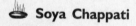

Soya Chappati

2 cups soya flour

1 cup wheat flour

Salt to taste

Mix together the soya flour, wheat flour and salt. Add enough water to make dough. Knead well. Make chappati without oil.

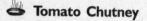

Tomato Chutney

2 big, ripe tomatoes, chopped

2 onions

1 flake garlic

4-5 sprigs coriander leaves

½ tsp red chilli powder

¼ tsp jeera powder

Salt and sugar to taste

Blend the tomatoes, onions, garlic and coriander leaves in a mixie.

Put this mixture in a non-stick pan, add chilli powder, jeera powder and salt and fry for about ten to twelve minutes until the water dries up and it becomes a solid mass. Serve hot or after chilling in the refrigerator.

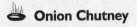 Kothmir Chutney

1 big bunch kothmir

4-5 sprigs of pudina

¼ ginger

2 flakes garlic

1-2 green chillies

Salt to taste

Blend all the ingredients in a mixie to form a chutney. You may add a pinch of sugar according to taste.

Onion Chutney

2 big onions, chopped

1 tsp channa dal

1½ tsp urad dal

½ tsp mustard seeds

2 dry red chillies

A bit of tamarind

Salt to taste

Heat a non-stick pan and put in the onions, dals and mustard and fry for two minutes. Then add the other ingredients and salt, and fry for four to five minutes. Remove the pan from the flame. When it cools, blend in a mixie to make chutney.

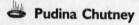 Pudina Chutney

1 bunch mint leaves

½ bunch coriander leaves

¼ ginger chopped

1 flake garlic chopped

2-3 green chillies

A bit of tamarind

½ tsp jaggery

3 tsp channa dal

2 tsp urad dal

½ tsp lemon juice

Salt to taste

Dry roast the dals till they are golden. Add all the other ingredients and make a paste in the mixie. Serve as chutney.

SALADS

Dal Salad (Kosambri)

¼ cup split yellow dal (moong)

1 cucumber, finely chopped

1-2 green chillies, finely chopped

5-6 sprigs coriander leaves, finely chopped

½ carrot, grated

1 tsp lemon juice

Pinch of hing

Salt to taste

Soak the dal for two hours. Add all the other items to the dal and mix well. Serve either chilled or at room temperature.

Tomato Salsa

4 ripe, firm tomatoes, peeled

6 spring onions (bulbs), chopped

1 green chilli

Chopped coriander leaves

1 tbsp lemon juice

½ capsicum

Salt and pepper to taste

1 flake garlic, crushed

Chop the tomatoes and capsicum into small bits. Add all the other ingredients and mix well.

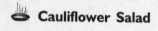

Cauliflower Salad

2 cups cauliflower, blanched (200 gm)

I tbsp coriander leaves

½ tsp jeera powder

½ tsp garlic paste

2 tbsp lemon juice

3 tbsp vinegar

Pinch of sugar

I green chilli, chopped

Salt to taste

In a pan combine the lemon juice, vinegar, chilli, sugar and garlic, and keep to boil. When it begins to boil add the jeera powder, coriander leaves and salt. Mix well. Add the cauliflower, mix well and leave on a low flame for a few minutes.

Mixed Vegetable Salad

2 cups mixed vegetables (beans, carrots, cauliflower, potato, etc.)

2 tbsp lemon juice

I tsp mustard paste

I tsp vinegar

½ tsp garlic paste

¼ tsp pepper powder

Pinch of sugar

½ tsp oregano (optional)

Salt to taste

Steam or parboil the vegetables. Mix together all the other items and add to the vegetables. Serve chilled.

Boiled Vegetable Salad in Curd

1 cup mixed vegetables, boiled (beans, carrots, sprouts, potatoes, etc.)

½ cup curd

½ tsp jeera powder

Chopped coriander leaves

1-2 green chillies

½ tsp mixed herbs

Pinch of salt and sugar

Mix all the ingredients except the vegetables well with the curd. Before serving, add the mixture to the vegetables and mix thoroughly.

Potato Raita

1 cup boiled and cubed potatoes

½ cup green gram sprouts

1 cup curd

I onion

I-2 green chillies

Chopped coriander leaves

Pinch of sugar

Salt to taste

Mix the curd with the onion, green chillies, coriander leaves, sugar and salt. Beat well. Add the potatoes and sprouts, and mix well.

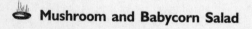 Sprouted Gram Salad

I cup sprouts (soak in water for one hour)

I onion

I green chilli

Chopped coriander leaves

I carrot, grated

I tbsp lemon juice

Salt to taste

Mix all the ingredients with the sprouts. You can add some ground pepper before serving.

Mushroom and Babycorn Salad

½ cup babycorn, parboiled

½ cup mushrooms

1 tsp lemon juice

½ tsp garlic paste

1 tbsp vinegar

½ tsp thyme

½ tsp oregano

½ tsp sugar

Pepper and salt to taste

Put all the ingredients in a non-stick pan. Cover and cook till it is dry.

🍲 Potato Channa Salad

1 potato, boiled, peeled and cubed

1 cup channa, boiled

½ cup sprouts (green gram sprouts)

1 onion, cubed

1 tomato, chopped

1 tbsp coriander leaves, chopped)

1 tsp mint leaves, chopped

1 green chilli, chopped

½ tsp jeera powder

3 tsp lemon juice

Salt to taste

Soak the sprouts in water for half an hour. Wash well. Mix all the ingredients together and serve immediately or chilled.

Cucumber-Sprouts Salad

1 cup curd, beaten well

½ cup sprouts

½ cup cucumber

¼ cup carrot

Mint leaves

Coriander leaves

¼ tsp garlic paste

¼ tsp jeera powder

½ tsp chilli powder

Salt to taste

Soak the sprouts in water for half an hour. Chop the carrots, cucumber, coriander and mint leaves finely. Mix all the ingredients with the well-beaten curd. Serve chilled or at room temperature.

Carrots in curd

1 cup carrot, grated

1 cup curd

1 tbsp coriander leaves

1-2 green chillies

½ tsp sugar

Salt to taste

Mix together the curd, green chillies, coriander leaves, salt and sugar. Add the grated carrot and mix well.

Potatoes cooked in curd

2 medium potatoes, boiled, peeled and cubed

I cup curd

I cup water

I tsp chilli powder

½ tsp jeera powder

I tsp coriander powder

I tsp sugar

Salt to taste

2 spring onions, chopped

Chopped coriander leaves

I green chilli, chopped

I tsp besan

Mix together the curd, water, chilli powder, jeera powder, coriander powder, sugar and salt. Let the mixture come to a boil over medium flame. While it is boiling, add the boiled potatoes, spring onions, green chilli and coriander leaves. Let it boil for five to seven minutes. Then add the besan mixed with one tbsp water. Let it boil till the gravy thickens.

Chapter 9

HEALTHY FOOD FOR THE HEART

Vegetables

ARTICHOKE

QUANTITY : One medium-sized artichoke

CALORIES : 53 calories

NUTRITIONAL VALUE: The vegetable contains moderate amounts of calcium, iron, phosphorus, niacin and vitamin C. It is also a good source of magnesium and potassium.

HEALTH BENEFITS: Artichoke is a valuable asset in your diet: the calcium it contains helps build your bones and teeth, iron enriches your blood, vitamin C wards off minor infections like cough and colds, and potassium keeps your blood pressure in check.

Go easy on artichoke if you are on a salt-free diet though; the has a very high sodium content.

Asparagus

QUANTITY: One cup of cooked asparagus

CALORIES: 44 CALORIES

NUTRITIONAL VALUE: Asparagus contains a winning combination of three essential, protective nutrients—carotene, the plant form of vitamin A, vitamin C, and selenium—in abundance. Together, they boost the body's immune system and form a formidable shield against cancer. Added to this are healthy doses of bone-building calcium, blood-enriching iron, phosphorus, cholesterol-lowering soluble fibres, and low fat and sodium levels.

HEALTH BENEFITS: An excellent diuretic. Eat plenty of asparagus to prevent kidney stones.

Beetroot

QUANTITY: 100 g cooked beetroot

CALORIES: 43 calories

NUTRITIONAL VALUE: Beetroot is rich in carbohydrates in the form of easily assimilable sugars, making it a supreme fuel food. It is a terrific blood regenerator, with its readily absorbable iron, and is the ultimate nourisher, with an abundance of vitamins (B, B2, B6, C and niacin), iodine, calcium and other essential minerals.

HEALTH BENEFITS: When you eat beetroot your body regenerates red blood cells quicker and maintains an optimum supply of oxygen to the cells, thus promoting a sense of great physical well-being. Eat plenty of it if you are anaemic. Beetroot juice is good for patients with hypertension and heart disease. It is a good laxative, though the juice, taken with a dash of honey, helps to control and reduce diarrhoea and nausea.

Bitter Gourd

QUANTITY: 100 g cooked bitter gourd

CALORIES: 25 calories

NUTRITIONAL VALUE: The tiny bitter gourd packs a rich cocktail of essential vitamins and minerals, especially vitamins A, B1, B2, C, and iron.

HEALTH BENEFITS: Bitter gourd is a good anti-pyretic appetizer and blood cleanser. But it really comes into its own in the diet of diabetics. The vegetable lowers sugar levels in the blood. To clean skin infections like itchiness, psoriasis, ringworms and so on, sip a cupful of fresh bitter gourd juice with a dash of lime juice on an empty stomach. You can also drink the juice to cure a hangover.

Brinjal

QUANTITY: 100 g brinjal

CALORIES: 14 calories

NUTRITIONAL VALUE: Its chief virtue is its total lack of sinful fat. It contains trace amounts of folic acid, vitamin C and fibre.

HEALTH BENEFITS: Funnily enough, nature did not endow this widely popular and bland vegetable with too much nutrition.

BROCCOLI

QUANTITY: One cup raw broccoli

CALORIES: 24 calories

NUTRITIONAL VALUE: Broccoli is so suffused with health and so tasty and versatile that it beats its cabbage patch siblings on the goodness scale. Broccoli has an abundance of carotene, which builds up your immune system and strengthens your eyes. It is a good source of calcium, and therefore great for children. It is rich in vitamin C, which protects you from minor infections, and has plenty of fibre, now acknowledged as the all-round health-maintaining agent.

HEALTH BENEFITS: Regular intake of broccoli may actually help lessen the risk of developing cancer and lower blood-cholesterol. It is an excellent addition to a diet for a healthy heart.

BRUSSELS SPROUT

QUANTITY: One cup cooked Brussels sprout

CALORIES: 55 calories

NUTRITIONAL VALUE: The Brussels sprout is dense with growth-assisting proteins, and has a richer concentration of it than most other vegetables. It is rich in vitamin C, the infection-fighter, and contains the ultra-nutritious, health-maintaining combination of vitamin A, riboflavin, iron, potassium and fibre. It also has low sodium and fat content.

HEALTH BENEFITS: The big news about Brussels sprout is that it is an active cancer-fighter, thanks to a substance called 'indole' which acts as a cancer-inhibitor.

CABBAGE

QUANTITY: 100 g cabbage

CALORIES: 27 calories

NUTRITIONAL VALUE: Nature's 'miracle vegetable' is crisp with health promoting and healing nutrients. It is the ultimate 'C' vegetable with generous amounts of calcium, carotene and vitamin C, which are all essential for every aspect of physical well-being. It is also believed to have anticarcenogenic properties. Added to this are generous amounts of proteins, phosphorus, iodine and fibre.

HEALTH BENEFITS: Juice from cabbage is a wonderful stomach cleanser, spiffing up the mucus membranes of the stomach. Raw cabbage juice contains an anti-ulcer factor, and is a great antidote for stomach ulcers. The roughage in cabbage makes it a good remedy for constipation. Eat chopped raw cabbage mixed with a little salt, black pepper and lemon juice for immediate relief from constipations. Nibble on raw cabbage leaves to stay slim—the tartaric acid in it inhibits the conversion of sugar and carbohydrates in the other food you eat into fat. Wrap a cabbage leaf blanched in boiling water around a sprained limb to relieve pain. For back pain, try this naturopath's remedy: boil a cabbage leaf in milk till it becomes a jelly, spread it on a cloth, apply over the affected area and leave overnight.

CURRY LEAVES AND CORIANDER LEAVES

NUTRITIONAL VALUE: Both coriander leaves and curry leaves are rich in proteins, vitamins and minerals. Coriander leaves are well-supplied with vitamins A, B1, B2, C and iron.

HEALTH BENEFITS: Added to your food, both coriander and curry leaves aid digestion. If you suffer from indigestion, try this remedy: add a couple of teaspoons of fresh coriander juice to a cup of buttermilk and drink it. The drink also helps reduce nausea. Mix a paste of curry leaves with buttermilk as an antidote for indigestion. Mix the juice of curry leaves with lime juice and sugar to stop nausea. Mash curry leaves with honey and drink the mixture as a syrup to stop diarrhoea. Apply a paste of curry leaves on boils and other skin irritations to soothe and heal.

CARROT

QUANTITY: 100 g carrot

CALORIES: 13 calories

NUTRITIONAL VALUE: In a cup of shredded carrot there is more than twice the amount of nutrients you would require for a day to build up your resistance to cancer and to strengthen your eyes. It contains carotene, plenty of vitamin C to checkmate the common cold, potassium to help your heart, and loads of pectin to lower your cholesterol level.

HEALTH BENEFITS: Take a daily swig of raw carrot juice, also known as 'miracle juice' to increase the secretion of digestive juices, strengthen your eyes, detoxify the blood, combat peptic ulcers, reduce symptoms of asthma and to generally keep the body in top condition. The juice, more than anything else, keeps your immune system fighting fit, and is a must if your immunity is down due to disease or medical treatment. A cupful of grated carrot gets rid of worms in the stomach.

Cucumber

QUANTITY: 100 g cucumber

CALORIES: 13 calories

NUTRITIONAL VALUE: Cucumbers contain potassium, sodium, magnesium, sulphur, silicon, chlorine and fluorine.

HEALTH BENEFITS: Keep cool with cucumber. It is an excellent body rehydrator, so eat lots of it, especially in summer, to restore electrolyte liquid balance in the body. Drink cucumber juice frequently through the day for immediate relief of hyperacidity of the stomach. Cucumber juice, in combination with carrot, beetroot and celery juices, is good for arthritis and rheumatism.

Cucumber is a natural diuretic, regulating your kidneys, while the roughage it contains aids bowel action.

Capsicum

QUANTITY: 100 g capsicum

CALORIES: 15 calories

NUTRITIONAL VALUE: One single capsicum will provide you with more vitamin C than a whole glass of the pure orange juice. Capsicum also contains bone-strengthening calcium and potassium.

HEALTH BENEFITS: Include capsicum, preferably raw, in your diet for a bagful of benefits, from warding off minor bacterial infections to putting the sparkle back in your eyes and skin, preventing tooth decay, aiding digestion and promoting healthy hair growth.

Ginger

NUTRITIONAL VALUE: Ginger enlivens your recipes, perks up your tongue, and best of all, goes to work on your body, cleaning, sprucing, toning and generally keeping you in glowing good health.

HEALTH BENEFITS: Chew on a small piece of ginger half an hour before a meal to sharpen your appetite and get the digestive system on the go. Chew it immediately after a meal to put an end to indigestion problems and nausea. If you find raw ginger too sharp on your tongue, chew sugar-coated pieces of ginger. To cure chronic indigestion, extract a teaspoon of fresh ginger juice, mix it with one teaspoon lime juice, one teaspoon mint juice and one tablespoon honey to make a syrup to be taken thrice daily.

To relieve a bad cold, boil a one-inch piece of ginger in a cup of water, strain, add a teaspoon of sugar and drink it hot. To reduce the cough which accompanies a cold, take a syrup of concentrated ginger mixed with honey. When you have a fever, boil fenugreek seeds in a cup of water, strain, add a teaspoon of ginger juice and a dash of honey, and drink it warm to bring down the fever and refresh the body. Add a piece of ginger to the water you use for making tea to refresh yourself during a fever. Pound dry ginger with a little water and apply to your forehead to relieve a headache. The paste relieves toothache when applied to the gums.

Ginger also helps you travel without feeling queasy.

Green Beans

QUANTITY: One cup cooked beans

CALORIES: 40 calories

NUTRITIONAL VALUE: Known as the French bean, broad bean or cluster bean, this stringy vegetable packs in a lot of punch. It contains a plentiful supply of blood-enriching iron, bone-strengthening calcium, and of course, the all-important fibre.

HEALTH BENEFITS: Pump up that iron in your blood with a daily dose of beans. Beans also strengthen your bones and teeth, and the high non-soluble fibre content regulates the bowels. Since they have little sodium and no fat, they are absolutely 'safe' for the heart.

Ladies Finger (Okra)

QUANTITY: 100 g okra

CALORIES: 17 calories

NUTRITIONAL VALUE: Okra has a high protein content. It is also rich in calcium, iron, magnesium and the vitamins A, B and C. Okra also has a high fibre content.

HEALTH BENEFITS: Okra has been thought to increase brain power, but nature has endowed it with other qualities as well. Like assisting the body's growth, strengthening and protecting bones and teeth, enriching the blood, helping the body absorb nutrients, and toning up the body's health-promoting mechanism.

Lettuce

QUANTITY: One cup raw lettuce

CALORIES: 10 calories

NUTRITIONAL VALUE: Cool crunchy lettuce is crisp with vitamin C, the general body strengthener and infection fighter, replete with carotene, which strengthens the eyes and inhibits cancer, and adequately endowed with blood-enriching iron and other minerals salts. It has absolutely no room for sodium, fat or carbohydrates—enough to take it to heart!

HEALTH BENEFITS: Soothe those jangled nerves and revv up that sluggish heart and liver with a bowl of lettuce. Raw lettuce is a must if you work out regularly, because it nourishes and revitalizes tired muscles. Drink a haemoglobin-boosting tonic of raw lettuce juice mixed with raw carrot juice, especially if you are slightly anaemic. For a good night's sleep, mix lettuce juice with rose oil and apply to the forehead and temples.

MINT

QUANTITY: 100 g mint

CALORIES: 48 calories

NUTRITIONAL VALUE: It refreshes, revitalizes and recharges you. It is actually a nutritive fiesta, with substantial amounts of growth-assisting protein, bone and teeth strengthening calcium, blood-enriching iron, vitamin C and phosphorus.

HEALTH BENEFITS: Add a few sprigs of fresh mint to the food you eat to aid in digestion. If you are down with indigestion, have a cup of mint tea. To make it, boil one teaspoonful of chopped fresh leaves in a cup of water, strain, add a pinch of ginger powder and sip. If stronger measures are needed, try this syrup—extract the juice of a handful of fresh mint leaves, add a teaspoonful each of lime juice and honey and drink frequently through the day. This syrup is also effective against threadworm infection and diarrhoea.

Mint has a therapeutic effect on the respiratory system. If you are on medical treatment for tuberculosis or asthma, add this juice to your daily diet: mix a teaspoonful of fresh mint juice with two spoons of pure malt vinegar and honey, stir into four ounces of carrot juice. Have it about thrice daily; it will nourish the lungs and boost the body's resistance to infection. Gargle with strong mint tea, to which a pinch of salt has been added, to soothe a sore throat and, as mint fans say, to sing with 'full-throated ease'.

Chew fresh mint leaves to prevent bad breath and tooth decay. Chewing fresh mint is also said to be a way of sharpening your taste buds. Sip a cup of mint tea with ginger before going to bed-it relaxes you and has a soporific effect.

ONION

QUANTITY: Two tablespoons chopped onions

CALORIES: 6 calories

NUTRITIONAL VALUE: The onion is rich in amino acids, essential for preventing heart disease. It abounds in vitamin A, which strengthens your vision and builds resistance against disease, calcium, which builds bones and teeth, and riboflavin, which enriches the blood.

HEALTH BENEFITS: A regular intake of onions, about two a day, in the opinion of the experts, increases 'good' (HDL) cholesterol and lowers 'bad' (LDL) cholesterol, which makes it an absolute must for people prone to hypertension and heart disease. The iron content in onions is easily assimilable, so the vegetable is good for keeping anaemia in check.

Added to this are its therapeutic properties. To get rid of a minor cough, mix equal amounts of onion juice and honey and take frequently, in teaspoonfuls, through the day. Chew a raw onion a day to keep the dentist away—the onion's bactericidal properties prevent tooth decay and disease. Follow that up with clove though, to remove the odour from your breath. To relieve toothache, place a small piece of onion on the tooth that is giving you trouble.

Peas

QUANTITY: One cup cooked peas

CALORIES: 134 calories

NUTRITIONAL VALUE: Peas have plenty of carotene, vitamin C, which combats minor infections, and the soluble fibre pectin, which is said to lower blood cholesterol. Nature's little giant gets even better with negligible fat and sodium content.

HEALTH BENEFITS: Peas are heart-friendly vegetables and can also be taken safely by diabetics. Externally applied, they have a soothing effect on itchy skin. Boil peas in clean water for a few minutes, strain, cool and apply to irritated skin for quick relief.

Pumpkin

QUANTITY: One cup mashed pumpkin

CALORIES: 48 calories

NUTRITIONAL VALUE: The pumpkin has exceptionally high fibre content. The vegetable gives you all-round nutrition too, especially carotene, the immune system booster and vision strengthener, and other essential minerals.

HEALTH BENEFITS: Pumpkin is an excellent body cleanser. Boil pumpkin seeds in water, strain, and drink to cleanse the blood and wash out the kidneys. Its high fibre content gets the bowels into shape. Pumpkin is especially good in the diet of people prone to hypertension and heart disease.

SAGE

NUTRITIONAL VALUE: Sage has quite a high vitamin A and C content but since only a few leaves are used for cooking the benefits is more medicinal than nutritive.

HEALTH BENEFITS: Season your dishes, especially those 'heavy' non-vegetarian dishes, with sage to aid digestion.

Feeling stressed out? Relax with a cup of sage tea: pour a cup of boiling water over a handful of chopped sage leaves, let it stand for a few minutes, then strain. Stir in a teaspoon of honey and sip it. The tea has a very mild sedative effect that calms overwrought nerves.

If you need to soothe a sore throat try this: pour half a litre of boiling water on a handful of sage leaves, cool, strain, add a little vinegar and honey, and use to gargle. Rub fresh sage leaves on your teeth and gums to keep them healthy and sparkling clean. You can also swill sage 'tea' around your mouth to reduce inflammation of gums and toothache. Soothe a tiresome allergic rash by dabbing on sage tea. Refresh yourself and hasten recovery from a fever with this sage drink: pour a litre of boiling water to a mix of 25 g sage leaves, 50 g honey and three tablespoon pure orange juice. Leave till it cools, then strain and sip it by the cupful. Fresh sage is also an antiseptic; strew a few leaves around the bed of a child suffering from measles.

SPINACH

QUANTITY: 100 g spinach

CALORIES: 17 calories

NUTRITIONAL VALUE: Deep green, succulent spinach is a great protein provider, containing more of the growth agent, in fact, than does an equal amount (in weight) of meat, fish, eggs and chicken. And it has the added punch of blood-enriching iron, disease-fighting vitamin A and haemoglobin stimulating folic acid. All without a hint of fat!

HEALTH BENEFITS: Increase the iron content in your blood with regular intake of spinach. And clean up those tissues and the digestive tract with nature's ultimate scavenger! Take an early morning drink of raw spinach juice mixed with carrot juice to stop bleeding gums and to get rid of mouth sores. Chew on spinach leaves to strengthen the gums.

SWEET POTATO

QUANTITY: One cup mashed sweet potato

CALORIES: 206 calories

NUTRITIONAL VALUE: A large amount of calories are packed into the sweet potato, but they are balanced with so much carotene—eight times your daily requirement in just one cup of mashed sweet potato, to be precise—that the vegetable ends up providing more value for the calorie content.

HEALTH BENEFITS: The carotene in sweet potato keeps your vision unimpaired and boosts your immune system. Some studies have shown that it lowers the risk of lung cancer, which means it is essential for you if you are a smoker. The starch present in it makes it a good fuel food which provides energy.

Fruits

APRICOT

QUANTITY: 100 g fresh apricot (three medium-sized fruits)

CALORIES: 53 calories

NUTRITIONAL VALUE: The apricot is full of carotene, the resistance builder and cancer-fighter, and is rich in potassium, which is good for the heart, haemoglobin-manufacturing iron and tissue-building copper. It is also highly energizing, containing lots of carbohydrates, though it has very little fat.

HEALTH BENEFITS: Apricot is just the fruit for you if are an active, outdoor kind of a person. Eat it as a pleasant medicine if you are slightly anaemic. To cool a body overheated by the sun or by fever, drink fresh apricot juice with a dash of honey.

BANANA

QUANTITY: One large banana

CALORIES: 116 calories

NUTRITIONAL VALUE: The banana is rich in growth-stimulating, high-grade proteins and energy-giving, easily assimilable sugars. To top it all, it is full of vitamin C, to ward off minor infections, and is entirely free of sodium, thus helping to lower blood pressure.

HEALTH BENEFITS: Eat a ripe banana and follow it up with a glass of milk for a quick, well-balanced, instantly energizing meal. Eat it to soothe an acidity-prone stomach and to ease constipation.

BERRIES

QUANTITY: Strawberries one cup, Raspberries one cup, Blueberries one cup

CALORIES: 45 calories, 60 calories, 74 calories respectively

NUTRITIONAL VALUE: Berries are not only the best desserts around, they are also good for your well-being. Strawberries, the most delicious of them all, contain, for instance, more vitamin C than an equal quantity of orange! Added to which they are rich in calcium, iron and magnesium.

All berries contain large amounts of non-soluble fibre and potassium-which makes them just the right kind of desserts for a healthy heart.

FIG

QUANTITY: 100 g fresh figs, 100 g dry figs

CALORIES: 80 calories, 274 calories respectively

NUTRITIONAL VALUE: Nature has loaded the temptingly tasty fig with energy-boosting sugars, large amounts of growth-assisting proteins, bone-strengthening calcium and plenty of fibre.

HEALTH BENEFITS: Snack on figs when you are low on energy and drive. They are the most effective natural laxatives. Figs work wonders on throat infections. To relieve hoarsensess and to banish bad breath, take fig syrup, made by soaking dried figs in water for a while and then stewing in honey. To soothe a sore throat, dilute one teaspoon of the syrup in half a cup of hot water, gargle with it and drink it.

Guava

QUANTITY: 100 g guava

CALORIES: 50 calories

NUTRITIONAL VALUE: This fruit should have been spelled with a C. Nature has endowed the deliciously soft mellow-yellow ripe guava with loads and loads of vitamin C, making it a prime health food. The guava also contains potassium, which should be good news for those with heart problems.

Grapefruit

QUANTITY: One large grape fruit

CALORIES: 74 calories

NUTRITIONAL VALUE: Grapefruit traps enough fibre, potassium, calcium and phosphorus to make it a valuable health food, just right for your heart, teeth and bones. And just a couple of fruits are enough to take care of your day's requirement of vitamin C, the infection-buster.

HEALTH BENEFITS: Get the digestive juices flowing with grapefruit juice, the great appetizer. The juice also spruces up your digestive tract. The fruit is a good addition to the diet of the diabetic.

Lime

QUANTITY: 100 g lime

CALORIES: 59 calories

NUTRITIONAL VALUE: A natural healer and beauty enhancer, sharp, tangy lime is nature's storehouse of citric acid, as also of vitamin C, calcium and phosphorous.

HEALTH BENEFITS: Start your day with a glass of warm water mixed with a teaspoon each of lime juice and honey to clean up the alimentary canal, stimulate secretion of digestive juices, slough off disease-causing bacteria, tone up the liver and work as a gentle laxative. Mix a teaspoon of lime juice and a pinch of sodabicarb in water and drink it to reduce acidity and ease indigestion. A teaspoon of honey mixed with a teaspoon of lime juice can stop vomiting and nausea. Rub squeezed out lime rind over your gums to reduce any swelling. Brush your teeth occasionally with salt-spiced lime juice to keep them sparkling.

Peach

QUANTITY: One medium-sized fresh peach

CALORIES: 50 calories

NUTRITIONAL VALUE: Pop a peach into your mouth and fill up on vitamin A to strengthen your vision and revv up your immune system. The fruit also contains vitamin C to ward off minor infections, and potassium which is beneficial for your heart.

HEALTH BENEFITS: Fresh peaches are great as much for what they don't have as for what they have. Low in sodium and fat and high in potassium, peaches are a healthy addition to any diet.

They also supply essential vitamins and mineral salts to keep body tissues and cells in top condition.

PINEAPPLE

QUANTITY: One cup chopped pineapple

CALORIES: 80 calories

NUTRITIONAL VALUE: Tough on the outside, all sweetness inside, the pineapple is one of those super foods that combine good health with great taste. The pineapple synthesizes proteins and carbohydrates thanks to the presence of an enzyme called bromelain. The fruit is also high on vitamin A, which is good for your eyes and your general immune system, and vitamin C, which keeps away the common cold. It also contains iron, magnesium and calcium.

HEALTH BENEFITS: Pineapple is an excellent dessert because it helps you digest your meal quickly and efficiently. Pineapple juice has long been considered an antidote to recurring colds and coughs. Drink a lot of the juice when you have a cold—it is much more effective than orange juice. Sip the concentrated juice to soothe a sore throat. Diluted pineapple juice refreshes you considerably when you have a fever and aids quick recovery. Since it is a 'concentrated' food, take it after or in between meals.

THE 52-WAY PATH TOWARDS PERFECT HEALTH

1. Start the day with a glass of warm water and a dash of lime.

2. Drink eight glasses of water a day.

3. Include two vegetables and one fruit in every meal.

4. Begin each meal with a raw vegetable salad.

5. Make a light snack of assorted sprouts.

6. Eat only fresh vegetables.

7. Once a week have only fresh fruits until noon; let your lunch be the first meal of the day.

8. Eat only freshly cooked meals, not refrigerated leftovers.

9. Include one green vegetable and one yellow vegetable in every meal.

10. Go on a 'juice fast' for a day. Start with vegetable juice, and sip fruit juice for lunch and dinner.

11. Kick the old coffee drinking habit. Have a glass of fresh fruit juice instead.

12. Avoid beverages like soda, coffee, colas and so on.

13. Cut out all deep-fried food from your diet.

14. Cut down on products like soft drinks, ice-cream, candy and cookies which have high sugar content.

15. Never skip a meal, even if you're on a diet. Eat a fresh fruit or drink vegetable juice instead.

16. Include foods with high fibre content—plenty of fruits, vegetables and grains—in planning your diet.

17. Use salt in moderation.

18. Wash vegetables thoroughly in clean water before chopping.

19. Steam or boil vegetables, rather than frying or sautéing them.

20. Retain peels of potato, cucumber, carrot and tomato while cooking.

21. Take a moment off to mentally list out the nutritional value of the food you're about to eat.

22. Don't rush through your meals. Set aside enough time to appreciate, enjoy and digest your food.

23. Make every meal an enjoyable experience. Set dishes out attractively and chew slowly to appreciate the full flavour of the food you eat.

24. Choose to be radiantly healthy. Keep yourself informed about the nutritive value of every food item you buy.

25. Shop for groceries yourself. Notice the look, feel and smell of fresh fruits and vegetables and enjoy their intrinsic goodness.

26. Watch out for eating habits paired with emotional states, like reaching for a chocolate when you're depressed. Resist the urge and eat fruit instead.

27. Eat popcorn (rather than chips) while watching a movie.

28. Sit at the table at meal times. Don't read the paper or review bills while eating.

29. Make it a point to have dinner with the entire family at the table, and not in front of the TV.

30. Eat just to the point when you are full. Don't stuff yourself.

31. Stop smoking.

32. Restrict alcohol consumption.

33. Get a good night's sleep, every night.

34. Enrol in an exercise programme today.

35. Take a brisk, twenty-minute invigorating walk each morning.

36. Spend ten minutes every morning and evening doing basic stretches.

37. Do not use elevators when you can climb the stairs.

38. Enrol in a transcendental meditation programme today.

39. Focus on your breathing. Take a deep breath, then exhale slowly. Repeat a couple of times a day.

40. Learn to relax. Spend twenty minutes consciously relaxing each muscle of your body.

41. Spend twenty minutes a day in silent meditation, prayer or contemplation.

42. Learn the healing power of laughter. Watch a crazy movie, recall a joke or read a funny book and laugh out loud.

43. Tap the powers of your subconscious. Relax your body for twenty minutes and project the 'Perfect You' in your mind.

44. Balance your lifestyle. Devote equal time each week to work and fun.

45. Join kids in a sports activity and rediscover the joys of childhood.

46. Keep in touch with friends. Call up or visit them and be at peace with the world.

47. Enrol in an activity like dancing, swimming or roller skating you never indulged in because you were afraid of 'what people might say'.

48. Forgive someone who you think has done you wrong and cleanse your spirit of rancour.

49. Do a something nice for someone you don't know too well, but who could do with a friend.

50. Spend a quiet half hour chatting with your family.

51. Listen to soothing music for at least fifteen minutes each day.

52. Read a good book once a week.

REFERENCES

Anand, B.K., G.S. Chhina, B. Singh. 'Some aspects of electroencephalograph studies in yogis.' *Electroencephalogram Clinical Neurophysiology* 13 (1961):452-456

Blackwell, B., S. Bloomfield, P. Gartside, A. Robinson, I. Hanenson, H. Magenheim, S. Nidich, R. Zigler. 'Transcendental meditation in hypertension.' *Lancet* 1 (1976):223-226.

Gardner, Howard. 1985. *Frames of Mind.* New York: Basic Book Inc. Publishers.

Goleman, Daniel. 1995. *Emotional Intelligence.* Bantam Books.

Joseph, S., K. Sridharan, S.K.B. Patil, M.L. Kumaria, W. Selvamurthy, N.T. Joseph, H.S. Nayar. 'Study of some physiological and biochemical parameters in subjects undergoing yogic training.' *Indian Journal of Medical Research* 74 (1981):120-124.

Manchanda, S.C., U. Sachdeva, K.S. Reddy, R.L. Bijlani, Dharmananda. 'Coronary atherosclerosis reversal potential of yoga life style intervention.' Ist International Conference on 'Yoga in Daily Life', 20-22 Dec 1996, New Delhi, Conference Handbook (Abstract).

Op.cit. 'Decreased blood pressure in borderline hypertensive subjects who practised meditation.'

Mihalyi, Csikzent. 1975. *Flow, the Psychology of Optimal Experience*. New York: Harper and Row.

Ornish, D., S.E. Brown, L.W. Scherwitz, J.H. Billings, W.T. Armstrong, T.A. Ports, S.M. McLanahan, R.L. Kirkeeide, R.J. Brand, K.L. Gould. 'Can lifestyle changes reverse coronary heart disease?' *Lancet* 336 (1990):129–133.

Salovey, Peter and John D. Mayer. 1990. *Imagination, Cognition and Personality*.

Telles, S., R. Nagarathna, H.R. Nagendra. 'Autonomic changes during 'om' meditation.' *Indian Journal of Physiological Pharmacology* 39 (1995): 418-420.

Udupa, K.N., R.H. Singh. 'The scientific basis of yoga'. *Journal of American Medical Association* 220 (1972):1365.

Wallace, R.K. 'Physiological effects of transcendental meditation.' *Science* 167 (1970):1751–1754.